To Phil
whose friendship I
so much appreciate,
and who has contributed
so much to my
professional development.

Asbjørn

Learning in Medicine

Edited by
Colin Coles and
Hans Asbjørn Holm

Learning in Medicine

Edited by
Colin Coles and
Hans Asbjørn Holm

Scandinavian
University Press

Scandinavian University Press (Universitetsforlaget AS)
0608 Oslo, Norway
Distributed world-wide excluding Norway by
Oxford University Press, Walton Street, Oxford OX2 6DP

Oxford New York Toronto Dehli Bombay Calcutta Madras Karachi
Kuala Lumpur Singapore Hong Kong Tokyo Nairobi
Dar es Salaam Cape Town Melbourne Auckland Madrid and
associated companies in Berlin Ibadan

Oxford is a trade mark of Oxford University Press

Published in the United States by
Oxford University Press Inc., New York

© Universitetsforlaget 1993

ISBN 82-00-21811-2

British Library Cataloguing in Publication Data
Data available

Library of Congress Cataloguing in Publication Data
Data available

Typeset by typer & tall, Norway

Printed in Norway by A/S Foto-Trykk, Trøgstad 1993

Table of Contents

Preface

In May 1991 a conference "Learning in Medicine" took place in Oslo. The Conference was organised by the Norwegian Medical Association, the University of Southampton, Medical Faculty, the Nordic Federation of Medical Education and the Norwegian Association of Medical Education.

This book is based on the proceedings from that Conference, but not only that, the dialogue between the authors and the editors has kept the process alive up to the very last editorial meeting. In fact, some of the keynote addresses at the conference, presented as chapters in this book, have been subject to quite radical changes, initiated by the authors themselves, reflecting the dynamics of the conference, the post-conference dialogue, and the influence of the activities which constitute our everyday life.

Acknowledgements

The editors want to thank the contributors to this book who responded so willingly and enthusiastically to our suggestions and did not in any way disappoint us in our expectations. We also want to express our gratitude to all the conference participants who have made their contribution by engaging in numerous discussions and dialogues, and thus facilitated in the process of clarification of issues along the road to a more comprehensive understanding of learning in medicine.

We also like to give very special thanks to Phil Bashook who, besides contributing significant chapters to this book, offered invaluable advice on the final editorial work and constructive criticism in the evolutionary process that led to the formulation of a theory of learning in medicine presented as the final chapter.

The Conference was generously supported by NYCOMED, Oslo, Norway.

Colin Coles
Hans Asbjørn Holm

1

The Oslo Conference

HANS ASBJØRN HOLM AND COLIN COLES

The conception and first draft of a conference

In a house in Southern England, one evening in early March 1990, two middle-aged men were sharing ideas about medical education, which filled most of their professional life.

Their road to medical education as a major area of interest had very different starting points, one with a background in educational psychology and the other in clinical medicine. It turned out, however, that they shared a strong discontent with much of what was labelled medical education and had very similar views on the guiding principles they thought should form the basis for medical education. They jotted down some notes, and out came a series of key phrases: learning is an individual process, you have to establish curiosity, it is about providing learning opportunities, content must be presented within a contextual frame, we learn best by reflecting on our practice, learning is both a cognitive and an emotional process, the teacher has a facilitating role, etc.

Next day the two sat on a Wessex Electric train to London enjoying each other's company and reaffirming and elaborating on the ideas that had filled them with such enthusiasm the night before. Then, shortly after the train had passed Woking, out of nowhere the idea of organising a conference with a focus on learning in medicine materialised and the planning started that very moment. They felt that the objectives of the conference and an outline of the format had to be discussed and agreed before they separated in London, one of them for a meeting, the other leaving the country. There was no time for hesitation. It seemed, however, that a lot had been going on on a subconscious level, and the conference took shape at a remarkable speed. By the time the train passed through Clapham Junction, a 20-minute ride from Woking, the objectives, as they later were presented to the invited people, had been settled:

- To allow those engaged in medicine to examine critically current understanding of the ways people learn
- To explore ways of applying this understanding in medicine, including
    - the full spectrum of medical education, from selection of undergraduates to lifelong continuing education
    - the full range of health care provision when the learner is the patient, client or the public
    - the provision of health care, in patient learning, in disease prevention, and health promotion
    - research issues, both in terms of basic research and applied research, that need to be addressed.

The organisation of even a small conference takes more than the enthusiasm of a couple of people. Fortunately, organisations with a strong commitment to medical education joined forces and made the conference come true.

The title of the conference, Learning in Medicine, replicated in the title of this book, was carefully chosen both to reflect the ideas of the organisers and to serve as a guide to the format of the conference. We wanted to promote a learner-centred approach in medical education, explore new avenues of implementation and practice, and examine if ideas inherent in learner-centred education could unfold and materialise within the conference format.

The conference

A short description of the conference will give some idea of the context in which the material published in this book was first presented, and how this fitted with our educational views.

To get a conference started the organisers first have to decide what the participants were likely to want from it. We wondered then if we could attract people simply by thinking up an attractive title, possibly adding some objectives, and by letting the participants decide the content and educational format. This we thought would be very much in line with a learner-centred approach.

In the preparation of Learning in Medicine we did not go that far, but as close as our courage took us. At the very least we thought that if the conference should benefit from the vast experience represented by the participants, a detailed time table filled with lectures would simply not do. Still we felt that just having people come to the conference, however dedicated to learner-centred education, without some sort of preorganised programme, could be too scaring both for the organisers and participants, and in the end really not serve the objectives of the conference. We settled for a programme that had some structure but plenty of opportunity for negotiating what would actually happen; these would as far as possible be discussed by the people who came.

The conference was a small one, just over fifty invited people met at the conference centre Soria Moria, located in a wooden scenic landscape in the mountainous outskirts of Oslo, a place especially suited to smaller, interactive, and contemplative, conferences.

The opening ceremony on Sunday May 12 introduced the participants to the art and life of the Norwegian painter Edward Munch. The last day of the conference was May 17, the Norwegian National Holiday, and the participants engaged in social activities the whole day. The organisers felt that building this into the conference was not without significance, beyond the fact that it gave us a good time.

The participants came from many parts of the world, although naturally Scandinavians formed the majority. Eleven countries were represented with nearly as many traditions in medical education. There was a good mix of medical doctors and educationists, and a smaller number of medical students who certainly represented the vigour and impatience of youth. In sum, the participants constituted a team of skilled and devoted experts in medical education, able to address in depth the full range of issues covering the acquiring and maintaining of professional competence.

What actually took place between May 12 and 17 is we hope reflected in this book. The final programme was a mixture of prescheduled events and participant-directed activities. A short plenary session each morning introduced important topics that constitute the major chapters of this book. Some of these had follow-ups in workshops that lasted as long as the participants felt feasible.

It is often hard to tell when learning actually takes place. We have often heard statements like "the most valuable part of the conference was sharing ideas with colleagues outside the lecture halls and group rooms". All the time spent in a conference should be valued, we felt, and in keeping with the best tradition of educational theory and practice, our emotional and physical needs must not be forgotten.

We tried to offer social activities that would nurture dialogue and creativity, exposing participants to art, museums, local culture and good food. Diversity of activities provides new forms of energy, enabling the participants to stand the hardships and challenges of another day's demanding workshops.

The conference process

The conference was thus characterised by a high degree of participant- and process-oriented activity, and this process has continued as the authors, in dialogue with the editors, have prepared their papers for publication.

Workshop topics had been suggested in advance in the invitation sent out several months ahead of the conference, but there was also a clear commitment to make changes as new topics emerged during the conference, which is indeed what happened. The participants were encouraged to suggest and organise workshops during the conference on topics important to them. But it was their own responsibility to attract participants. Towards the end of the conference the organisers felt that the participants really had taken a significant leadership role in the conference, that the conference had reached a substantial degree of self-directedness. To a very large extent it had been participant-centred, and we the organisers mere facilitators of the process.

The process of "letting go" is not always easy to face for those responsible. It might create, however unwarranted, a feeling of being out of control, and that chaos would ensue. That might, of course, be deleterious to the productive social texture of the occasion which could be broken into pieces. Alternatively, too, forcing people into workshops and group activities, might create a sense of coercion which would also be counterproductive to the learning process.

We feel that these challenges were reasonably addressed and that the processes were not overly disruptive or disposed. To keep the participants informed of what was going on outside their "own world", and thus enabling them to change track as ideas emerged and met others, afternoon plenary sessions were held where people gave short reports on the day's workshops. In addition, the participants could read about the various activities in a conference newspaper which was published daily and available at breakfast each morning.

The atmosphere and the processes going on during the conference are naturally difficult to convey in writing to people who were not there, and yet we feel that if we could do so adequately it would be a key to unlock the messages contained in this book. The conference certainly gave us a lot to reflect on, both related to the content of the various keynote addresses and the workshops, and not least important the insight into the very process of learning which emerged from the conference topics and the process of the conference itself. That we have tried to do in this book but perhaps inevitably we have found it difficult to achieve. Perhaps the conference process is best summed up in Rogers' well known phrase "Freedom to learn".

For the editors the conference was an important event in a process leading up to the final chapter: Learning in Medicine: Towards a Theory of Medical Education. We hope the book will provide the readers with enough input to decide for themselves if the editors' ideas make sense or not in the world the readers know.

How the book is arranged

The published papers represent a broad scope of educational topics. They may be viewed as elements of an educational mosaic which the editors have tried to fit together and present in an order intended to create a logical process. They may, however, very well be read separately, and the book as such may serve as an educational handbook on aspects of learning in medicine.

The various chapters are not necessarily published in the order they were presented at the conference. Some participants were invited to present keynote addresses. After the conference they were asked to reflect upon them and make appropriate revisions in the light of their conference experiences. Their ideas were submitted to the editors who gave their response before a final draft was completed. Other participants held workshops, some of which we felt were of such general significance that they should be more formally written up and presented as chapters here.

These *conference papers* are organised in four themes, each containing two chapters. This section of the book clearly demonstrates the manifold dimensions of learning in medicine. The fourth theme, chapter 9, reminds us of the eternal values and joy of reading and writing in the learning of medicine, and the need to broaden our scope to take a wider view if medicine is to survive as a humanistic discipline.

Following the conference papers the *workshops* are listed and ideas and thoughts pertaining to them are presented to the reader.

The workshop reports are duplicated exactly as they were reported in the conference newspaper the following morning. They can only give a taste of what went on and do not in any way pretend to convey the atmosphere or processes taking place which simply cannot be conveyed, and the chapter by Coles and Bashook attempts to say why. Duplicates of the workshop reports may serve, however, to give a more complete picture of the themes that were highlighted during the conference and thus help readers identify some important features of the conference.

The editors had some initial ideas that made them want to organise such a conference with a focus on learning in medicine. The conference process, the planning, the conference itself and the time spent working with the material that emerged from it, all have been important events in the process that led us to formulate our *Theory of Medical Education.* This final chapter likewise attempts to draw together the threads running through the book which we think summarizes and synthesizes the ideas and experiences that were exposed and explored at the Oslo Conference during five very eventful and significant days in May 1991.

Theme 1

Lifelong Learning and Continuing Medical Education

The two papers in this theme describe a continuum of ideas about how medical students and practitioners function in their daily activities as adult learners. Both papers provide a detailed literature review that in many respects has common origins in the thinking of William Osler and Donald Schön: one writing at the turn of the last century, the other at the end of the present one. Paradoxically their ideas have a lot in common but then perhaps the ideas are themselves timeless.

The purpose of developing skills in lifelong learning is to equip the physician with the skills and competencies to continue their own self-education beyond the end of formal medical training. Continuing medical education is one means by which physicians can do this. These two papers describe these important learning processes. The paper on lifelong learning provides a theoretical and practical basis for positing that medical schools and residency training programmes must help students develop the habits and skills and reflective attitude essential to becoming self-directed in their learning. The paper on continuing medical education broadens the definition of CME beyond classroom style programmes to include self-directed learning to gather information and reflection, and reviews the literature on information searching behaviour of physicians' within the social context of CME. It concludes with an endorsement of the theory of physician learning and behaviour change based upon a careful study of physicians' actual learning behaviour undertaken by the Society of Medical College Directors of Continuing Medical Education in the United States.

2

Lifelong Self-directed Learning: A Critical Ingredient of Medicine as a Profession

PENNY JENNETT

Introduction

Medicine as a *profession* traditionally represents the mastery of a specialised, theoretical body of knowledge, and the application of this knowledge in practice. It also embodies experiential knowledge, the skills therein, and the resultant art, wisdom, and intuition which belong to the profession (1,2) Both features evolve and flourish through the ongoing act of *reflection and renewal*, a skill depicted by Sir William Osler, a renowned physician and *lifelong learner*. Because the skills of reflection and lifelong renewal are not explicit, they are often not cultivated and emphasized either in the socialisation and training of future physicians, or in the understanding of practice itself (1, 2, 3).

The purpose of this paper is to describe why the professional acts of reflection and renewal inherent in self-directed, lifelong learning are critical to keeping up-to-date with respect to the mastery of theoretical knowledge; and, central to developing and nurturing experiential knowledge and the artistic "know how" of practice. Implications for curriculum, teaching, and designing learning opportunities will be offered, along with examples of applications.

Self-directed learning enables the learner to incorporate new experiences, to relate present situations with previous experiences, and to reorganize current experiences based upon this process. Self-directed learning is a reflective act of practice (4,5). The need for self-directed lifelong learning skills in medicine is emphasised by examining the traditional and experiential components of the profession through the work of Cervero (6). Schön (5), and Nowlen (2).

First, Cervero (6) notes the importance of both declarative (abstract, formal, and general) and procedural (specific, based in practice, practical) knowledge (Figure 1). He indicates that the

Cervero (1990)

Traditional	Broader
Declarative Knowledge	Procedural Knowledge
- abstract	- specific
- formal	- based in practice
- general	- practical
"knowing something is the case"	"know-how" "intuition" "art"

both play a role

Figure 1

former is "knowing that something is the case," and the latter is "know how" and "intuition". Declarative knowledge provides the ability to generate new knowledge and approaches, and permits sense to be made of practical knowledge. It provides the underlying principles and regularities which can re-shape practical knowledge. Both abstract knowledge and practice knowledge are required to develop and improve wisdom and wise action. The latter requires ongoing reflection and renewal based on involvement in practice. Schön (5) presents a parallel perspective. He sees professional learning as consisting of two dimensions: 1) structured knowledge, and reflections on this knowledge and associated acts within a given situation, and 2) ideas, exchanges, events, tactics, and examples brought to the situation for subsequent reflection, the professional "inner voice" or "art". The two components act in concert (Figure 2). Intuitive judgement, skills, and a "feeling" for a situation evolve through practice and reflection on it. Formal knowledge is brought to an event and reflected upon, but practice reveals a "kind of know-ing" which does not stem from prior individual knowledge. The professional is able to adjust to particular situations and produce new actions by adopting a reflective inquiry. Self-education and renewal result.

Nowlen (2) also indicates that the profession consists of basic knowledge and skills. As well, the professional and the patient are embedded in many cultures (family, religious, civic, recreational, educational, and occupational) in which professional meaning and professional growth take place (Figure 3). The professional, the

Schön (1983)

Dimension #1   Dimension #2

- Structured knowledge   – Ideas, exchanges, events
- Reflections on   brought to a situation
  knowledge and acts   for reflection

                                                "inner voice" or "art"

                     two dimensions act
                         in concert

Figure 2

environment, and the patient are continually evolving. Practitioners therefore must develop understandings and self-managed learning skills to recognise and adapt to the influence of these cultures.

Cervero, Schön, and Nowlen recognise and value the traditional, theoretical knowledge base; the art and the craft of the profession; and the need for continuous renewal based upon reflective experience. Respect for these dimensions has implications for learning across the continuum. These implications will be discussed under three sub-sections: 1) curriculum, 2) teaching, and 3) learning.

Nowlen (1988)

Dimension #1   Dimension #2

Basic knowledge and skills   Cultures (family, religious,
                                                civic, recreational, educational,
                                                and occupational)

                                                Professional meaning and
                                                personal growth take place

Figure 3

Lessons for curriculum

Schön (5) views learning as a "continuous, reflective conversation or dialogue with *practice*." Cervero (6) notes the importance of modelling *learning* from *practice*. With this background in mind, four perspectives on curriculum are offered. Nowlen (2) indicates that formal educational experiences must be positioned within larger self-directed frameworks (Figure 4). Cervero (6) reports that formal knowledge must be integrated into professional repertoires of professional knowledge and reasoning; the latter consisting of images, examples, scenarios, and practical principles (Figure 5). Schmidt

IMPLICATIONS FOR CURRICULUM

Nowlen (1983)

Formal educational experiences must be
positioned within larger self-directed frameworks.

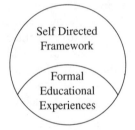

Figure 4

IMPLICATIONS FOR CURRICULUM

Cervero (1990)

Formal knowledge must be integrated
into practical knowledge.

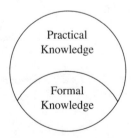

Figure 5

et al. (7) in their work addressing experts/novices, also outline the importance of practice and experience to move students and practitioners appropriately through the stages of knowledge, development and use. It is through the reflective process of self-renewal, self-directed learning, and experience that the skills of pattern recognition develop, and the professional begins to recognise both the element of surprise and variations on the norm.

McGuire (3), at a more basic level, notes curriculum to be much broader than content, in that it includes the total educational environment. She quotes from the Edinburgh Declaration World Federation of Medical Education (8), which emphasises the need for a society-based education which incorporates items such as: 1) the process by which information is acquired, 2) self-directed and interactive learning opportunities, 3) patient-based, ambulatory teaching, 4) ongoing linkages between medical education and the health care delivery system, and 5) managerial and leadership responsibilities. These five points are directly linked to reflection, renewal, and learning which respond to practice, society, or community needs.

Teaching

This curriculum approach requires a different perspective on *teaching* with a major re-focus on the responsibility of the teacher to guide the learner to question, to reflect, and to acquire self-directed learning skills. The teacher must also act as role model for these skills. The following quotes pick up this central theme.

"If he (teacher) is indeed wise he does not bid you enter the house of his wisdom, but rather leads you to the threshold of your own mind."
                                             – Kahlil Gibran, *The Prophet*

"The critical point of the process of teaching – learning is how the learner is aided to embark on this active, growing, changing, painful, or exhilarating experience we call learning."
                                             – Kidd, 1976

"There is a distinction between being at the leading edge of medicine and being able to teach medicine in order to foster the creation of strong anchor points in the students' memories on which their future experiences can be built."
                                             – Bordage, 1987

How does a teacher design optimal learning experiences to enhance this process?

Learning opportunities

Schmidt (13) Houle (1) Gibbons et al. (14) Schön (5) and Fox et al. (15) provide us with guidance as to what types of learning opportunities will facilitate learning, as well as cultivate the critical skills of lifelong learning. Specifically, Schmidt (13) suggests that learning environments should involve scenarios which encourage students to: 1) pull on prior knowledge so that they can hook current knowledge onto prior knowledge, thereby permitting the use of information stored in long-term memory, resulting in better understanding and better retention, 2) act in contexts which closely parallel or resemble a situation in which information may be applied, thereby permitting the "coding specificity", which adds to meaning and memory, and 3) elaborate upon information (e.g. note taking, responding to questions, discussing information with peers and teachers, teaching others, and formulating and criticising hypotheses) facilitating redundancy, and therefore remembrance and efficient recall.

Houle (1) provides guidance as to how students can be encouraged to develop effective learning skills. He outlines that students should be given learning opportunities which cultivate the development of confidence in their ability to learn and in their points of view, to set realistic goals and measure their accomplishments against these goals, to actively fit new ideas and new facts into context, to feel comfortable in seeking help and support when required, and to consciously learn beyond the point necessary for immediate recall. Gibbons et al. (14) have similar views in that they believe students need to engage in learning situations which permit them to internalise control over their learning; move toward their individual goals; develop originality, uniqueness, and integrity; work cooperatively with other team members and disciplines; and to identify themes in their individual lives which they can build on to create new ones. Future physicians and practitioners need to develop skills to accommodate information processing, as opposed to information memorisation; work in small groups to appreciate group dynamics and the value of other perspectives; and take responsibility for designing their own learning experiences.

Schön (5) and Fox et al. (15) pick up on Gibbons' point that students must develop self-education habits. Schön (5) emphasises the need for future and current practitioners to adopt an ongoing reflective, critical inquiry (research in practice) to discover relationships and identify "gaps". This process requires modelling the unfamiliar on the familiar, and results in a re-framing of questions around the unexpected. It requires an openness which exposes situations to public enquiry and leads to growth. Learning opportunities which promote self-confidence, question asking and reflection, openness and risk taking, uncertainty and surprise are therefore encouraged.

Bordage (11), in his study of long-term memory, indicates that students and practitioners can best learn around highly representative prototypes which act as "anchor points for the remainder of members in a category". These prototypes have the greatest number of features (e.g. symptoms, signs, pathophysiological characteristics, etc.) in common with other members of the category. In addition, borrowing from Rosch's 1976 work (12), he points out that there are three levels of concept abstraction (general, intermediate and specific), and that students learn best focusing upon the intermediate level of abstraction (e.g. "general level – Ischaemic disorders; intermediate level – angina pectoris; specific level – Gairdner's disease").

We now can ask even more practical questions. What specific applications and skills can facilitate the development of these lifelong learning habits?

Skills and applications

Let us re-focus for a moment and return to the definition of self-directed learning and its characteristics:

> "A dynamic process in which the learner reaches out to incorporate new experiences, relates present situations with previous experiences, and re-organizes current experience based upon this process."
>
> – Knowles, 1975

> "A central part of self-directed learning is the reflective act of practice."
>
> – Schön, 1983

Three examples of applications which are now currently being used in learning environments to cultivate such skills of self-directed learning and reflection are: the use of simulated patients, the integration of peer and self review, and the adaptation of Medical Informatics tools. Each application will be addressed briefly.

The use of simulated patients is now an activity cultivated in many medical schools. If used correctly as both a learning and evaluation tool, it fosters learning by providing contexts which resemble practice situations, thereby increasing meaning and memory. This learning process, however, will not foster self-directed learning habits critical to the ongoing maintenance of competence unless the principles of instructional design, previously offered by Schmidt, Schön, Fox, Bordage, and Houle, are followed.

Despite the recognition and importance of self and peer review in the practice of a profession (i.e., the need and ability for a professional to objectively and consistently evaluate one's own professional performance against oneself and others), activities to foster these skills often fail to be incorporated across the continuum to permit future and current physicians to comfortably experience and practice this activity (16,17,18,19). Goldfinger (20) in his *New England Journal of Medicine* editorial, "The Case for Contamination", notes that repetition and validation, two integral elements of these processes, are essential components of a physician's effective learning. This "contamination", Goldfinger states, is crucial as a stimulus to the process of further learning and professional development.

Medical informatics tools, such as those for searching and critiquing bibliographic data bases; the use of computer-assisted learning (CAL) and expert systems; patient and physician data bases; and electronic mail and bulletin boards, provide opportunities to practice skills associated with information management, sharing and critiquing. These skills are central to fostering the habits of reflection and renewal required for the ongoing maintenance of competence. These habits, as a stethoscope, become part of the tool box of practice.

Summary

This paper, by moving from the theoretical to the practical, emphasises why self-directed learning as defined by Knowles (4) is a critical skill for future and practising physicians. Implications for curriculum, teaching, and learning have been offered, along with the mention of specific applications.

Self-directed, continuous learning, and its inherent skills (Figure 6), is not an isolated activity. On the contrary, it is a dynamic process.

To develop and foster the habits, the professional must recognise self-identified learning gaps and act responsibly upon them. Furthermore, professionals must practice these habits on an ongoing basis. Students, teachers and medical education administrators must recognise the need for medical students and professionals to cultivate these skills across the continuum.

The art, practical knowledge, and expertise of medicine are lasting characteristics of the profession which adapt to professional, community and societal needs. The reflective, self-directed student and practitioner will best meet the dynamic and flexible needs of the profession of medicine today and in the future.

LIFELONG SKILLS/HABITS OF LEARNING

- recognise and deal with uncertainty, complexity uniqueness, and value conflict

- define problems, as well as solve problems

- professional and self renewal skills
  - "research in practice"
  - practice reflection
  - raise searchable questions from learning
  - openness

- fill the self-identified "gaps"
  - information seeking, critiquing, and sharing medical informatics tools

- optimise the "fit" between profession, organisation, government and other disciplines
  - society and community-based practice
  - medical resources

- partake spontaneously, and with comfort, in peer and self review
  - practice profiles, audits, feedback

- Address society's changing needs and expectations
  - cultural sensitivity
  - value sensitivity
  - multi-disciplinary team care

Figure 6

I close with these quotes from Osler (21).

"The hardest conviction to get into the mind of a beginner is that the education upon which he is engaged is not a college course, not a medical course, but a *life* course, for which the work of a few years under teachers is but a preparation."

"The most hurtful thing the practitioner can do is to fail to realise, first, the need for a lifelong progressive personal training and, secondly, the danger lest, in the stress of practice, he sacrifice that most precious of all possessions, his mental independence."

References

1. Houle CO. Continuing Learning in the Professionals. San Francisco: Jossey-Bass, 1980.
2. Nowlen PM. A New Approach to Continuing Education for Business and the Professions: The Performance Model. New York: MacMillan, 1988.
3. McGuire C. The Curriculum for the Year 2000. Med Educ (1989); 23:221-27.
4. Knowles M. Self-directed Learning: A Guide for Learners and Teachers. New York: Association Press, 1975.
5. Schön DA. The Reflective Practitioner: How Professionals Think in Action. New York: Basic Books, 1983.
6. Cervero RM. The Importance of Practical Knowledge and Implications for Continuing Education. Journal of Continuing Education in the Health Professions 1990; 10:85-94.
7. Schmidt ITG, Norman GR, Boshuizen HPA. A Cognitive Perspective on Medical Expertise: Theory and Implications. Acad Med 1990; 65:611-21.
8. Report of the World Conference on Medical Education. Edinburgh: World Federation for Medical Education, 1988.
9. Axford RW. Adult Education: The Open Door to Life-long Learning. Indiana, PA: The A.G. Halldin Publishing Co, 1980.
10. Kidd JR. How Adults Learn. New York: Association Press, 1973.
11. Bordage G. The Curriculum: Overload and too General. Med Educ 1987; 21:183-8.
12. Rosch E, Simpson C, Miller RS. Structural Basis of Typicality Effects. J Exp Phychol [Hum Percept] 1976; 2:491-502.
13. Schmidt HG. Problem-based Learning: Rationale and Description. Med Educ 1983; 17: 11-16.
14. Gibbons M, Bailey A, Comeau P, Schmuck J, Seymour S, Wallace D. Toward a Theory of Self-directed Learning: A study of experts with formal training. Journal of Humanistic Psychology 1980; 20:41-56.
15. Fox RD, Mazmanian PE, Putnam RW. Changing and Learning in the Lives of Physicians. New York: Praeger, 1989.
16. Linn BS, Arostegui M, Zeppa R. Performance Rating Scale for Peer and Self-assessment. British Journal of Medical Education, 1975; 9: 98-101.
17. Engebretsen B. Peer Review in Graduate Education. NEJM 1977; 296: 1230-121.
18. Fuhrmann B, Weissburg M. Self-Evaluation. In: Morgan M, Irby D (eds). Evaluation of Clinical Competence in Health Professions. St. Louis, Missouri: Mosby, 1978.

19. Louis A, Willoughby TL, Calkins EV. Self-Evaluation in Undergraduate Medical Education: A Longitudinal Perspective. J Med Educ 1985; 60:21-8.
20. Goldfinger SE. The Case for Contamination. NEJM 1982; 306:540-1.
21. Osler W. Aequanimitas and Other Addressed to Medical Students, Nurses, and Practitioners of Medicine (2nd edition). Philadelphia: Blakiston, 1906.

3

Clinical Competence and Continuing Medical Education: Lifelong Learning to Maintain Competence

PHILIP G BASHOOK

Physicians are self-directed learners. They decide what to learn, when to learn it, and how to learn it. Physicians learn what they want to learn to maintain competence. Participating in continuing medical education (CME) programmes is one of many ways physicians stay current or obtain information needed in managing a particular patient problem or clinical situation. As part of post-graduate medical education the term "continuing medical education" as used here is the time period in a physician's career after formal training (medical school and residency or registrar) and until retirement from medical practice when physicians function as practitioners. CME programmes can be part of a physician's efforts to gather or search for information to help in decisions about referring a patient for care, consider alternative ways of planning care for a class of patients, or restructure one's practice.

CME is not just pre-planned courses and conferences. In the broadest sense CME includes self-directed learning activities like reading, computer-aided self-study programmes, self-assessment tests, and even searching one's personal library or in a medical library for information. Physicians frequently use informal means to gather information. Some common methods are: consulting with colleagues (commonly referred to as hallway conversations), learning from conversations with industry representatives (i.e. pharmaceutical companies, medical equipment manufacturers, suppliers), listening to patients, and watching videotaped medical programmes.

During medical school and residency training most physicians develop lifelong habits for acquiring new knowledge (1). As self-directed learners physicians are constantly struggling with the problem of sifting through the explosion of new information and the irrelevant and frequently erroneous published reports of new discoveries. They develop personal learning styles to cope with the avalanche of information, but sometimes the sifting task becomes overwhelming.

CME programmes can provide one means of sorting out the essential knowledge from extraneous flotsam. Few, if any physicians I have met, will acknowledge they have resigned themselves to limit their search for information. The medical education challenge is to develop better ways to help the physician as a self-directed learner become an efficient and effective lifelong learner that assures him or her of maintaining clinical competence. The research literature on continuing medical education, physician behaviour in searching for information, and adopting medical innovations offers useful insights about how to change the continuing medical education enterprise to enhance clinical competence for self-directed learners.

This chapter will address a number of issues relating continuing medical education to clinical competence through lifelong learning. First, there will be an exploration of the concept of CME and provide a definition encompassing more than just pre-planned courses. In this discussion also are considered two important aspects of physician behaviour: what is known about how physicians search for information; and what is known about how physicians adopt new innovations into their practices that result in changing their practice behaviour. Next will be a consideration of clinical competence and how it is evaluated. In the United States, for example, accreditation of medical training and the assessment of physicians has been developed to satisfy even the most consummate bureaucrat. Finally, there will be a discussion of the linkage between CME, clinical competence, and lifelong learning with the goal of maintaining competence.

Continuing medical education as classroom instruction

Continuing medical education is part of a pattern of activities undertaken by physicians to maintain competence over their lifetime. Abraham Flexner, the famous progressive educator who evaluated American and Canadian medical schools in 1910 (2) and European medical schools in 1912 (3), summarised in one sentence what some consider the role of CME: "the post-graduate school was originally an undergraduate repair shop." (2, p. 174). For some physicians this may still be true, but nearly all, in the USA at least, continue their formal medical training by completing residency training in a specialty (97 % according to the Association of American Medical Colleges (4)), and many take additional subspecialty fellowship training. Continuing medical education in today's context begins after formal training in residency or fellowships. For most physicians CME is lifelong learning to maintain competence.

The traditional idealised portrait of CME resembles classroom instruction in grade schools. It begins with physicians participating in a course, workshop, or conference with the specific intent to learn something they plan to use in practice. This portrait assumes a teacher-centred approach to learning using the following reasoning: both the physician and the CME programme planners know and agree upon the physician's needs; the physician selects a CME course because of a wish to gather specific information for direct application in patient care; the CME course contains the appropriate learning opportunities in palatable form with ample opportunities for the physician to be nourished by information and experiences; the physician takes the nourishment home and applies it directly to the next appropriate patient; and, lastly there is evidence that what the physician has applied can be seen as a change in the patient's health status.

This is an idealised portrait because it is not real. Few doctors go to CME courses, conferences and workshops because they have a definite and burning desire to learn something they plan to use in practice immediately after taking the course. From this small cluster of physicians an even smaller number are at the stage of adopting an innovation to be ready to use the acquired information with patients. Even for these doctors there are concerns about practical matters that are best learned by informal conversations with colleagues.

Most physicians attend CME programmes to hear what new developments are being considered by experts, talk to colleagues about these developments and any other relevant topics, and explore how their own knowledge compares to what others consider current and relevant (5). Rarely, if ever (less than 5%), do doctors attend CME courses with the specific intent to learn how to change behaviour. We should be concerned about any physician who attends a course without prior preparation and immediately decides to change behaviour. Such physicians may be too willing to adopt new behaviour without first carefully weighing the benefits and problems.

Another problem with this idealisation of traditional CME is that most CME programme planners do not design the courses with the necessary specific information or experiences that doctors can translate directly for use in practice. Some breakout sessions (e.g. workshops and small group discussions) may offer a few experiences of this kind, but most CME programmes are designed as one-way communication: from the expert to the physician learner. The expert communicates what the expert wants the audience to know, not necessarily what the physician participants need or want. In the jargon of education it is "teacher-centred" not "learner-centred;" it is as if doctors are being treated like children in a classroom teaching.

Continuing medical education as self-directed adult learning

This chapter began with a statement about physicians as self-directed learners. Physicians are also adult learners in the classic sense described by Alan Knox (6) and Malcolm Knowles (7). Robert Richards (8) has conceptualised CME for adult learners in a way that includes the formal courses and conferences and the informal self-directed activities adults employ in learning. He portrays CME as an iceberg (Figure 1). The upper and smaller part of the iceberg, that part visible to most observers, is controlled by teachers, CME faculty. Typical CME programmes in the "visible CME" include courses, conferences, workshops, hospital-based symposia and lectures, and individualised instruction (e.g. self-assessment examinations, audiovisual programmes, computer-aided programmes). These "visible CME" activities are only a small part of the iceberg of CME activities used by physicians as self-directed learners.

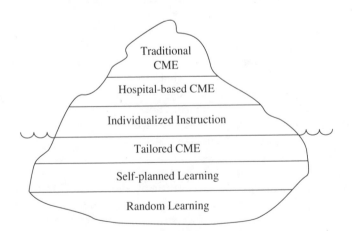

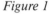

Figure 1

Below the water line are the more significant and greater number of self-directed learning opportunities that occur most frequently for physicians. For example, learner-centred CME can be informal or random learning from "hallway consultations", or perusing the medical journals and other medical literature for interesting articles. It can be self-planned learning when a physician decides to contact an expert for advice, or the physician reads the literature on a disease or patient situation. Tailored CME fits into informal CME when a physician assesses his/her practice and plans a personal CME programme for specific experiences to learn new behaviours. Gullion and colleagues at the University of California, San Francisco (9) and Sivertson, Meyer and colleagues (10) at the University of Wisconsin in Madison developed self-directed learning for physicians beginning with practice appraisals.

Richard's CME iceberg (fig. 1) helps in understanding how to link CME and clinical competence. Physicians as self-directed learners pick what they want to learn, search for the best means of learning it (formal courses, tailored CME, etc.), and decide when and where they plan to learn it. With the needed information and experience they decide how to use it for their practice and to assure their personal maintenance of competence.

Reading as an important information source

A number of studies have considered how physicians search for information and select the best source for the information. Not surprisingly, for most physicians reading is the primary means used to acquire new information (8). Studies done in Canada point to reading either from journals or one's personal library as the first place physicians look for new information (11,12).

Manning and Denison (13,14) studied what sources physicians used to adopt two new medical innovations that very few had learned during their formal training. The innovations were new to medicine at the time of the study: echocardiography and cimetidene. They found that cardiologists read reports in journals as their primary information source to learn about echocardiography, a diagnostic procedure (13). Eighty-one per cent had not heard of echocardiography before this time. The most popular source for internists to learn about cimetidene, a new generation of medications for ulcer disease, was by reading journals (14). However, physicians do not necessarily receive the information in a timely way because it may not be published in the journals they read.

As an example of this problem one study assessed how primary care practitioners (family physicians and internists) who treated diabetics obtained information about photocoagulation for diabetic retinopathy (15). They found 46 % of the family physicians and 60 % of the internists knew of a major multi-centre clinical trial on photocoagulation, but only 28 % of the family physicians and 46 % of the internists knew the study results. Variables like number of diabetic patients and being board certified in the specialty had little effect on the findings.

The most important finding from Stross and Harlan's study came from their assessment of the availability of the clinical trial findings in the medical journals most often read by primary care practitioners. Clinical trial results had been published two years earlier in the *American Journal of Ophthalmology*, but only some letters to the editor had been published in the journals read by the primary care practitioners. It is not surprising that so few of the physicians had learned about this important study for the management of diabetic patients. Also, it should not be surprising that these physicians had not adopted photocoagulation treatment of diabetic retinopathy as recommended in the clinical trial. If they were to be judged about maintaining competence in treating diabetic patients, should their performance be considered inadequate?

Reading also plays an important role in the daily lives of physicians as noted by studies about how many hours most physicians read medical literature. Studies about physician reading habits, going back as far as 1955, suggest the typical physician reads medically related material between 4–5.5 hours per week (8). Many physicians report that they read medical literature for pleasure. On a personal note, when I asked the family physician who was my doctor for the first 17 years of my life, he reported he considered reading medical literature his private time and a way to relax. Now he is over 80 years old and continues to read the literature although he limits his practice to a few days a week.

Reading is not the sole or primary information source for all situations. Which information source is selected first or second depends on the purpose of the search. The typical doctor may search for information or new knowledge with different motives in mind (16). When faced with a pressing patient problem the most common approach is to consider "what is the fastest, cheapest and easiest way for me to learn what I want to know?" (17). Studies of information searching behaviour find different patterns to the search process depending upon what physicians wish to learn and their medical specialty.

Another study by Stross and Harlan (18) on dissemination of findings from two major multi-site reports on hypertension, the Veterans Administration Cooperative Study (VA) and Hypertension Detection and Follow-up Programme (HDFP), demonstrated 40 % of family physicians were aware of the VA and HDFP findings and 80 % learned about them from medical journals. After six months 63 % of the internists knew of the VA and HDFP findings with 97 % aware of the results; 40 % learned of the findings from CME courses. The difference between the results of this study and Stross and Harlan's study of photocoagulation can be explained by two facts. These hypertension studies were disseminated rapidly in the journals the primary care practitioners read most frequently, rather than first published only in specialty journals. The second reason is that sponsors of CME programmes were aware of the studies and quickly developed or incorporated the findings into courses for primary care practitioners.

The studies by Manning and Denison (13,14) referred to earlier, also shed light upon how information sources are useful to become aware of new medical developments and how these sources help physicians learn to use the new findings in practice. In both studies physicians used multiple sources of information. The echocardiology study (13) found that 49 % of the cardiologists' first information source to become aware of the procedure was printed matter (journals, books, throwaway material), 21 % looked to meetings and conferences, 7 % to colleagues, and 6 % to CME courses. In contrast to learning about the procedure, 42 % of cardiologists learned how to perform it from reading printed matter, 22 % from CME courses, 17 % from meetings and conferences, and 4 % from colleagues. The emphasis on learning how to perform the procedure shifts slightly away from self-directed learning using printed matter to participation in pre-planned programmes (37 % learning from participation in meetings, conferences and courses).

In the study on learning about cimetidine (14), physicians were asked to rank order all information sources they used to become aware of the medication, and how they learned about using it. Physicians reported obtaining critical information on cimetidine preferentially from medical journals, then CME programmes, and thirdly physician colleagues. This was also true for learning how to manage patients on the drug.

Physician communication and adoption of medical innovations

Understanding how physicians interact and adopt new drugs, procedures, diagnostic techniques or treatment plans has long been of interest to medical sociologists. There are two thrusts to the investigations. One approach looks at the communication networks among physicians and attempts to understand how information is disseminated from primary sources to physicians and among physicians. A second approach investigates how individual physicians adopt innovations new for use in practice.

1. Communication networks among physicians

The grandfather of studies on dissemination of information among physicians was done by Coleman, Katz, and Menzel (19). They investigated the dissemination of information about a new antibiotic among general physicians in Columbia, Missouri. They found clusters of physicians in touch with each other and diffusion begins from an inner circle of physicians who are early adopters to a wider circle who wait until the innovation has become more established by their peers. Also, some physicians serve as "gatekeepers" and provide the local medical community an immediate expert judgment on the usefulness of recommended innovations.

Stross and colleagues in Michigan investigated how the communication networks are involved in practitioners' adoption of new diagnostic and treatment methods for rheumatoid arthritis (20), osteoarthritis (21), and pulmonary disease (22). They identified physicians who functioned as gatekeepers in local medical communities and determined that many of the physician "gatekeepers" were local colleagues others turn to for advice and information. These physicians were not specialists in the specific disease topic but colleagues others trusted and could obtain information from in a straight forward and understandable manner.

The "gatekeepers" functioned as "educational influentials" (EIs), something like a professor in residence but without a formal title or responsibilities (23). The studies by Stross and colleagues attempted to train the EIs about the various disease areas, let the EIs disseminate the information to their colleagues in the community as they felt appropriate, and measured the impact of this "CME intervention". They carefully assessed changes in practice and new knowledge acquired by the local physicians after a reasonable time interval. This series of studies demonstrated that the EIs do communicate the new knowledge through informal communication networks, the local physicians do change behaviour, and the EIs appear to be a key source of influence in changing physician knowledge and behaviour.

Informal communications between physicians has been studied previously and typically occurs as "hallway" consultations, telephone conversations about patients, or at breaks in CME programmes or conferences (24,25).

In one study I participated in, we investigated the informal communication networks among internists and family physicians in five local practice communities (26). We employed as the intervention CME programmes on diabetes mellitus that focused upon adoption of new diagnostic nomenclature and diagnostic techniques. We found three separate informal communication networks of physicians that sometimes interconnect through a few physicians common to each network. One network was composed of physicians on the full-time medical staff of a hospital. Most physicians in this network were board certified specialists. Their communication style involved equal two-way communication among specialist colleagues.

Another network was composed of physicians on various hospital staffs but as volunteers with a full-time independent private practice. Most of these physicians were general internists or family physicians. These physicians communicated among themselves only in small clusters of three or four when they had shared office space or were partners in a practice. They communicated in one direction, to the hospital-based physicians, particularly the specialists, by obtaining consultations on their patients. The office-based physicians did not receive reciprocal communication from the hospital-based physicians except as reports on the individual patients.

The third group of physicians were isolated from the other networks and generally worked in solo office-based practices. They seemed to be separated from the wider medical community not only in their limited communication with colleagues, but their infrequent participation in medical conferences at the hospital or local medical schools. In essence these physicians were really individual isolated practitioners who had limited communication with anyone and did not employ formal CME programmes as a social contact or opportunity to gather information. Friedson (27) labels these individuals "social isolates" of the medical community. It is difficult to assess whether they were able to maintain their clinical competence through informal CME activities. My hunch is that these are the individuals many CME programmes target and most planners of CME programmes fail to attract to the conferences.

2. Physician adoption of innovations

The literature on adoption of innovations by physicians is less extensive than studies on communication networks. Geertsma studied the physicians' adoption of innovations by developing a hypothetical model based upon a series of pilot studies (28). They tested the model by applying it to a random sample of 66 physicians from five specialties. The four stages in the model are: *Priming* – the physician feels dissatisfaction with some aspect of his practice behaviour; *Focusing* – the physician becomes aware of alternative or new practice behaviour; *Rationalisation* – the physician envisions solutions to any practical problems associated with the potential change; *Triggering* – the physician responds by implementing a change after a clear communication regarding the desirability of the change; and *Evaluation* – after making the change the physician assesses the practical result.

In Geertsma and colleagues' validation of the model they were initially concerned that some of the physicians would not have made practice changes or recall what they did. In fact, using one-hour follow-up interviews after physicians completed a lengthy questionnaire the investigators found most physicians wanted to report on many more changes than time permitted. The investigators found differences in use of the stages depending upon the type of change reported (diagnostic technique, use of new drugs, administrative practices, etc.). Colleagues (37 % of reported instances) were the most influential in the focusing stage of change followed by journals (34 %) and hospital conferences (18 %). CME programmes played a much less important role and accounted for only 5 % of the focusing stage influence. Physicians' follow-up activities (triggering and evaluation stages) were most influenced by colleagues (47 %), with journals (32 %) still very important but conferences (9 %) and CME programmes (9 %) of lesser value.

The Maxwell study (26) referred to previously found results similar to the Geertsma study in five hospital-connected physician communities addressing adoption of new approaches in diabetes. One important finding added to the Geertsma study was that the complexity of the innovation to be adopted became important in physician decisions to use information sources and in how the physician approached the challenge of changing behaviour.

For example, some innovations were easier to adopt such as switching from prescribing an established medication that required close patient monitoring for side effects to a newer medication with fewer detrimental side effects and less need for patient monitoring. Adopting the newer medication is reasonably easy for two reasons: first and foremost is the fact the physician retains control over the prescribing process and does not have to rely upon other health professionals to assure patient compliance; and second because the newer medication eliminates a concern for accurate information from the patient about serious side effects and the need to perform laboratory tests to titer the dosage. Hard to adopt innovations in the Maxwell study appeared to be situations in which the physician had less control over the treatment process and forced the physician to rely on others for effective patient management. For example, diabetic care frequently involves referring patients to diabetes teaching services, which place control of the situation out of the hands of the physician. In the Maxwell study of diabetes care some physicians hired nurses and trained them to perform the appropriate tasks under the supervision of the physician. In both studies (26,28), the knowledge needed for these changes was available from a variety of sources.

Clinical competence and practice

A number of authors have defined clinical competence for use in assessing physicians. Burg and Lloyd (29) analyzed the various definitions of clinical competence and recommend a framework for defining competence that includes functions a physician must perform in providing care to patients in specific clinical situations. Using their framework most definitions distinguish between competence and performance and describe the assessment of competence as assessing both knowledge and performing abilities. Performance assessment entails looking at samples of actual practice to establish the capability of physicians to use what they know in specific clinical situations (30).

The best measures of clinical competence come from a comprehensive assessment of a physician's knowledge base and representative samples of performance with patients including measures of the outcomes. During medical training most medical schools, hospitals and training programmes assess clinical performance daily and usually on every patient seen by a student or resident/registrar.

Knowledge is less often assessed and usually by informal means during case presentations or hallway or hospital corridor discussions about specific diseases or patients. For physicians in practice clinical competence is assessed only periodically and usually only when a physician obtains a license to practise medicine or volunteers to be evaluated by peers during specialty board certification programmes administered by national certification organisations (e.g. Royal College of Physicians and Surgeons in United Kingdom, Member Boards of American Board of Medical Specialties in USA).

At a less direct level and definitely removed from day-to-day physician practice are surrogate measures of a physician's actual competence using a review of credentials. In the United States, Great Britain, most Commonwealth Countries, most countries in Europe, and other countries following the Germanic or British medical education traditions and health care models there are three ways physicians can demonstrate their competence to the public through their credentials: certification in a specialty or subspecialty, licensure to practise by a state, province or territory, and obtaining hospital privileges to be on the hospital medical staff.

The variations in using credentials as surrogates for assessment of performance occur as a spectrum of possibilities. At one extreme are the complicated and patchwork systems in the United States involving federal and state government regulations, financing of hospital and physician care by private and public sources, hospital accreditation requiring medical staff review of individual physician's credentials, accreditation of CME programme sponsors, 54 separate medical licensure boards, and 24 separate primary specialty certifying boards.

In contrast, a more cohesive system exists in some European countries and the United Kingdom as well as many other developed countries to assess clinical performance and competence. Most countries employ a cooperative centralised plan developed jointly by governmental agencies, the medical community, physician certifying organisations, and organisations representing the public. The Norwegian system involving the government and Norwegian Medical Association is a typical example.

Another perspective on competence can be garnered from asking physicians what they consider as competence. It is the high personal standards that physicians set for themselves that defines personal competence and how closely they met the standard according to Putnam and Campbell (31). "The desire to excel" or "do one's best" are reasons individual physicians reported for changing their performance. An individual physician's standards may be similar or different from other physicians' depending on a variety of factors including: the patient care situations the physician encounters, a need to express excellence beyond one's colleagues' expectations, and a grasp of the body of knowledge and skills considered essential for competent practice.

The latter issue, physicians wanting to be sure about the grasp of knowledge and skills, frequently drives participation in formal CME programmes. CME participation becomes converted from a learning opportunity to a measure of competence through designating credit hours for participation and offering recognition awards for attendance at accredited CME programmes. The hours and the awards have little to do with learning and are questionable measures of competence.

Linkage between lifelong learning CME and maintaining competence

The linkage between lifelong learning, CME and maintaining clinical competence has not been well investigated except for one study (The "Physician Change Study" (32)). Most published studies use experimental research methods that assume learning is a discrete event (i.e. the CME programme intervention) and change in observable practice behaviour or finite knowledge are the measurable variables. Even employing experimental research methodology (which may have questionable value for investigating many sociological phenomena) in some published accounts of the impact of preplanned CME programmes on practice have demonstrated limited, but definite positive effects (33,34,35).

A number of reviews of the published literature criticise the quality of the evaluation studies, especially the lack of control groups in experiments (36). The few reviews using meta-analysis statistical techniques to evaluate studies of CME impact on practice support the claim that physicians will change behaviour as a result of participating in pre-planned CME programmes, if two conditions are met: the programmes are carefully designed, and the impact measures are carefully drawn. Sanazaro (37) reviewed the literature on CME and improving competence. He suggested that CME can make a difference in the ability to provide good care. However, he also points out that CME does not necessarily result in habitual and consistent competent performance.

Absent from the literature are studies demonstrating connections between self-directed CME and maintaining competence (38). One study used a non-theory based clinical trial experimental format to assess the impact of self-directed CME on practice (39). Although published in a prestigious medical journal, the methodology was too flawed to provide valid conclusions. The study had one significant and unexpected outcome. It was one of the factors that served to galvanise the Society of Medical College Directors of Continuing Medical Education, a professional association of physicians and non-physician educators responsible for CME programmes in US and Canadian medical schools, to begin a seven-year qualitative and descriptive research study on how physicians change and learn (The "Physician Change Study" (32)).

The "Physician Change Study"

The "Physician Change Study" was begun in 1982 by a core group of medical educators from the Society with the intent of understanding from the physician's perspective how physicians change their practices and lifestyles and how learning was involved. Initially they hoped to provide only a description of change and the role of learning, but the final report includes a well-developed theory of change and learning by physicians. I think this study is clearly on the right track to understand the role of CME in lifelong learning. It certainly supports my views about the role of CME in physician practice changes and resonates with my bias toward more descriptive research before investing in theory-based clinical trial-type experiments.

The Society members contacted physician colleagues, arranged a one hour face-to-face interview in the physician's office or other work setting, and used a semi-structured questionnaire format to capture "stories about changes" undertaken in their life or practice. The semi-structured interview format followed the traditional social anthropologic methodology outlined by Dexter when performing specialised interviews to obtain in-depth information (40).

Twenty-three interviewers collected change stories from physicians located throughout the USA and Canada. A sample of 775 usable cases from 340 physicians remained (2.2 cases per physician on average) after unusable cases were eliminated. The physicians studied were a reasonably representative sample useful for comparison with other studies investigating the change process of practitioners. Although the data were not collected as critical incidents, the investigators used the data analysis methodology of critical incidents to develop and validate categories and conceptual structures that explained the case studies. The conceptual structures and summaries of the data form the results and provide the empirical foundation for a theory on change and learning. Separate chapters discuss various aspects of how physicians change in their lives and their practices.

The "Physician Change Study" combines elements of qualitative methodology from different traditions and conflicting paradigms (education, sociology, anthropology, and medicine) to create a report that generates the theory. As such, the report "findings" represent an extension of the actual data collected in the interviews, but enriched and intermixed with the investigators' interpretations and conclusions. Key assumptions include suppositions that are reasonable and supportable by other work on change and inno- vations. For example, "People do not alter themselves or their lives arbitrarily – they have reasons;" "Changes are not automatically achieved." "Changes may range from the minor (grudging acquies- cence) to the all-encompassing (changes of career, lifestyles, and relationships)" (32, page 6).

The report concludes with a theory of learning and change that is supported by excerpts from the interviews. The theory posits that forces for change take the form of personal, professional and social forces or combinations of these three forces that can be represented in a Venn diagram (overlapping circles) (Figure 2). "Professional and personal forces are more likely than social forces to lead to learning as a means for change," according to their findings (32, page 164).

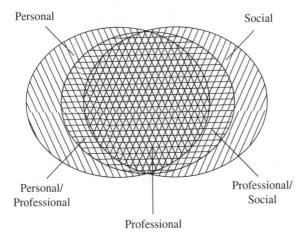

Figure 2 The interrelationships of forces for change

A second component of the theory addresses dimensions of learning in the change process. They propose linkages between forces for initiating change and using learning as a means to change. For example, problem-specific learning was associated more with professional and social forces for change, and conceptually-oriented learning was associated more with social forces for change.

Further refinements include the role of clarity in change either to clarify the characteristics of the forces for change or the potential kind of changes being made. Learning sometimes was helpful to clarify a problem but was more often associated with solving concrete problems than with broadening conceptual understanding. Types of changes were defined in the model as "incremental" small and simple changes, "adjustments" in one's life or practice, and "redirection or transformation" of significant and complex elements of one's life or practice. Learning had different but predictable associations with the forces for change and the types of changes.

Combining these elements of their theory produces a process of change and learning with four key components (Figure 3): 1) forces for change (personal, professional, social) which are directed through a prism in the physician's thinking to clarify the causes and/or visualise effects of a change; 2) a clarification process that generates a clean and clear image of the future change and helps direct thinking about the role for learning in the change process; 3) a decision process that uses the discrepancy between the physician's perceived current knowledge/skills assumed to be needed to reach the visualised goal and what skills must be acquired to achieve the goal; and 4) through personal effort the physician initiates learning activities, which may include CME, to acquire the skills or knowledge needed or initiates a re-assessment of existing knowledge/experiences with the intent of making a change (32, page 172). The theory does not address directly how long the change process can take except to imply a time frame by the "types of changes" and examples used to elucidate "incremental" changes, or "redirection" and "transformations." The physician interviews did not address the time variable except to ask the length of time for learning.

The theory does not describe how CME events fit temporally into the change process. They propose that pre-planned learning occurs in a rational sequence following introspection and clarification of discrepancies in an individual's knowledge/skills with what is expected to be necessary to make a change. This "rational thought process" becomes automatic upon repetition and is reminiscent of John Dewey's treatise in 1938 on *Education and Experience* (41). My hunch

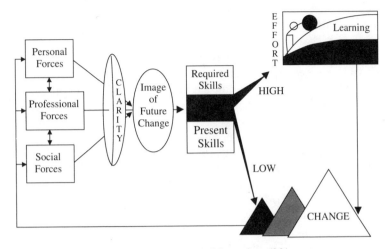

Figure 3 The process of change and learning (32)

is that "problem solving" learning occurs this way, especially for "incremental" changes. For "adjustments" and "re-direction" the process of change is much more complicated and I suspect there is a recycling and intermixing of planned and serendipitous learning events that influence change decisions and actions. Geertsma alludes to this idea with his explanation of recycling the change process through his four steps (28).

Overall, the "Physician Change Study" offers a refreshing description and analysis of physician learning and a proposed theory of how physicians change and use learning in the change process. The study provides a valuable contribution not only because they build upon empirical findings from the interviews, but because the theory can generate testable hypothesis to resolve some of the perplexing discrepancies found in published experimental studies on the impact of CME programmes.

Summary

In reviewing the research literature on continuing medical education it is interesting to note the way CME programmes have been interpreted by many to mean only formal classroom instruction. However, physicians recognise they are adult learners and self-direct to what they wish to know and learn, but the CME enterprise, at least in most developing countries, has been slow and reluctant to acknowledge that fact. Challenging this traditional conception of CME is Richard's Iceberg. It offers a way of conceptualising CME that combines traditional classroom instruction and self-directed CME into a personal plan for lifelong learning. I tend to subscribe to Dr. Richard's Iceberg because it visualises CME as the full range of learning activities that physicians draw upon during a life-time of learning.

Adding to the Iceberg conception in my vision of CME is the research on CME that demonstrates the importance of knowing how physicians search for information and adopt innovations. Physicians do not change behaviour in discrete increments which can be measured pre- and post-CME programme intervention. CME is more than discrete learning events; it is a part of a social phenomena. Moreover, in my view CME does not cause changed behaviour; CME is one of the activities physicians undertake as they attempt to maintain either their personally defined competence or standards set by others.

The "Physician Change Study" highlights a number of factors that resonate with my thinking about CME, lifelong learning and competence. I concur with their description of forces for change as the motivation for engaging in learning. Also helpful is distinguishing between different types of changes from incremental to significant transformations of lifestyle and activities. Using their theory one could construct a simple mathematical equation to explain a change process that begins with a notation (variable A) for the forces of change followed by a notation (variable B) for the type of change, followed by a notation (variable C) for the statement of clarity and learning, followed by the physician's decisions (variable D) about what needs to be learned, a separate notation (variable E) on how it will be learned, and ending with a notation (variable F) on the evidence of what changes have been made. I doubt there is a linear relationship among these variables, but empirical studies certainly could elucidate their relationship. Comparable equations could be developed to describe learning events for a number of physicians, or the same physician over many years. Over a lifetime there might be thousands of equations for a single physician. It is likely patterns would emerge from studying these equations that would be helpful in understanding individual learning styles, and the role of CME in lifelong learning.

In conclusion I will not be presumptuous and propose what CME should look like given what is known today about this enterprise. We have come a long way from Flexner's criticism of "post-graduate medicine as the undergraduate repair shop". This review of CME, I hope, provides the reader with a convincing explanation for CME as more than pre-planned classroom instruction; CME is part of a complex process of change, social interactions, and learning which physicians undertake to maintain competence.

References

1. Manning PR, DeBakey L. Medicine Preserving the Passion. New York: Springer-Verlag, 1987.
2. Flexner A. Medical education in the United States and Canada. A report to the Carnegie Foundation for the Advancement of Teaching. New York: Arno Press, Bulletin #4, (Reprint Edition, 1972), 1910.
3. Flexner A. Medical education in Europe. A report to the Carnegie Foundation for the Advancement of Teaching. Boston: D.B. Updike, The Merrymount Press, Bulletin #6, 1912.
4. Association of American Medical Colleges. AAMC Annual Report. Washington, D.C.: The Goetz Printing Co., 1991.
5. Cervero RR. Factor analysis study of physicians' reasons for participating in continuing education. Journal of Medical Education 1981;56, 29-34.
6. Knox AB. Teaching adults effectively: New directions for continuing education. San Francisco: Jossey-Bass, 1980;74-101.
7. Knowles M. Self-directed learning: A Guide for Learners and Teachers. New York: Association Press, 1975.
8. Richards R. Physicians' self-directed learning: A new perspective for continuing medical education, I. Reading. Mobius, 1986; 6(2):1-13.
9. Guillon DS, Adamson E, Watts MS. The effect of an individualized practice-based CME program on physician performance and patient outcomes. The Western Journal of Medicine 1983;138(4):582-8.
10. Sivertson S, Meyer T, Hansen R, et al. Individual physician profile: Continuing medical education related to medical practice. Journal of Medical Education 1973;48:1006-12.
11. Curry L, Putnam WR. Continuing medical education in maritime Canada: The methods physicians use, would prefer and find most effective. Canadian Medical Association Journal 1981;124:563-6.
12. Lockyer JM, Parboosingh JT, McDougall G. et al. How physicians integrate advances into clinical practices. Mobius, 1985;5:5-12.
13. Manning PR, Denson TA. How cardiologists learn about echocardiography: A reminder for medical educators and legislators. Annals of Internal Medicine 1979;91:469-71.
14. Manning PR, Denson TA. How Internists learned about cimetidine. Annals of Internal Medicine 1980;92:690-2.
15. Stross JK, Harlan WR. The dissemination of new medical information. JAMA 1979;241:2622-44.
16. Richards R. Physicians' self-directed learning: A new perspective for continuing medical education, II. Learning from colleagues. Mobius, 1986;6:3:1-7.
17. Hummel LJ. Unpublished doctoral dissertation. East Lansing, Michigan, 1985.
18. Stross JK, Harlan WR. Dissemination of relevant information on hypertension. JAMA 1981;246:360-2.

19. Coleman J, Katz E, Menzel H. Medical Innovation: A Diffusion Study. New York: Bobbs-Merrill, 1966.
20. Stross JK, Bole G. Continuing education in rheumatoid arthritis for the primary care physician. Arthritis and Rheumatism 1979; 22:77-81.
21. Stross JK, Bole G. Evaluation of an educational program for primary care practitioners on the management of osteoarthritis. Arthritis and Rheumatism 1985;28:108-11.
22. Stross JK, Hiss R, Watts C. et al. Continuing education in pulmonary disease for primary care physicians. Annual Review of Respiratory Diseases 1983;127: 739-46.
23. Hiss R, MacDonald R, Davis W. Identification of physician educational influentials (EI's) in small community hospitals. Proceedings of the 17th Annual Conference on Research in Medical Education: Association of American Medical Colleges, 1978.
24. Rogers E, Shoemaker F. Communications of Innovations. New York: The Free Press, 1971.
25. Wenrich J, Mann F, Morris W. et al. Informal education for practising physicians. Journal of Medical Education 1971;46:4.
26. Maxwell J, Bashook PG, Sandlow L. The role of communication networks in physicians' adoption of innovations. Proceedings of the 23rd Annual Conference on Research in Medical Education: Association of American Medical Colleges, 1984.
27. Friedson E. Professional Dominance: The Social Structure of Medical Care. New York: Aldine Publishing Co., 1970.
28. Geertsma RH, Parker R, Whitbourne S. How physicians view the process of change in their practice behavior. Journal of Medical Education 1982;57:752-68.
29. Burg FD, Lloyd JS. Definitions of Competence: A conceptual framework. In: Lloyd JS and Langsley DG, editors. Evaluating the Skills of Medical Specialists. Evanston, IL: American Board of Medical Specialties, 1983.
30. Bashook PG, Bordage G, Curry L, Guilbert JJ, Newble D, Pendleton D, Tunnell R. How to assess competent physicians: The issue of competence v. performance. In: Wakeford R, editor. Directions in Clinical Assessment: Proceedings of the First Cambridge Conference, Churchill College, Cambridge, England, June 25-July 1, 1984. Cambridge, England: Cambridge University School of Clinical Medicine, 1985.
31. Putnam RW, Campbell MD. Competence p.79-98. In: Fox RD, Mazmanian PE, Putnam RW. Changing and Learning in the Lives of Physicians. New York: Praeger, 1989.
32. Fox RD, Mazmanian PE, Putnam, RW. Changing and Llarning in the Lives of Physicians. New York: Praeger, 1989.
33. Davis DA, Haynes R, Chambers L, Neufield V, McKibbon A, Tugwell P. The impact of CME: A methodological review of the continuing medical education literature. Evaluation and the Health Professions 1984;7:251-83.
34. Bertram D, Brooks-Bertram P. The evaluation of continuing education: A literature review. Health Education Monographs 1977; 5:330-62.
35. Lloyd JS, Abrahamson S. Effectiveness of continuing medical education: A review of the evidence. Evaluation and the Health Professions 1979;2:251-280.
36. Lloyd JS. Hospital Privileges and Specialty Medicine. Evanston, IL: American Board of Medical Specialties, 1986.
37. Sanazaro PJ. Determining physicians' performance: Continuing medical education and other interacting variables. Evaluation and the Health Professions 1983;6:197-210.
38. Haynes R, Davis DA, McKibbon A, Tugwell P. A critical appraisal of the efficacy of continuing medical education. Journal of American Medical Association 1984;251:61-4.

39. Sibley JC, Sackett DL, Neufeld V, et al. A randomized trial of continuing medical education. New England Journal of Medicine 1982;306:511-5.
40. Dexter LA. Elite and Specialized Interviewing. Evanston, Illinois: Northwestern University Press, 1970.
41. Dewey J. Education and Experience. New York: MacMillian Company, 1938.

Theme 2

Faculty as Teachers and Counsellors

In the first theme we saw how professionals develop through continuing medical education, and that this rests on people directing their own learning. This presupposes, of course, that they know how to go about this. The second theme shows how young professionals need guidance in their training, and describes attempts to teach senior clinicians how to provide help to their juniors to achieve this.

The two papers under this heading deal then with the important roles of doctors, as teachers and counsellors. Doctors take on the teacher and counsellor role in many settings without necessarily being assigned a formal position where these duties are evident. This applies when teaching students and trainees, and also when dealing with patients. Many doctors also are in the position where counselling in relation to the public, directed towards politicians or public officers of many kinds, is part of their daily work. Also, during the last decade, the role and competence of doctors as leaders have been strongly challenged. Doctors certainly have to take on leadership. They should be encouraged to do so and offered training to meet the challenge. The art of counselling and mentorship are skills that are needed to exercise professional leadership.

Chapter 4 discusses training medical teachers to teach, and emphasises the importance of the teacher/learner relationship in continuing medical education. It argues the case for a learner-centred approach to medical teaching, and describes an example from the United Kingdom where consultants are being trained as "educational supervisors". The model used is then applied to a number of informal and formal teaching situations.

Chapter 5 describes a very similar situation in Norway where consultants are trained to undertake a role which is being called "educa-

tional counselling". This has remarkable parallels with the work described in Chapter 4 with "educational supervisors". Although there are some differences between the interpretation of the words "counsellor" and "supervisor", the general principles appear much the same. The Chapter emphasises the importance of trainee doctors being helped by their consultants to see for themselves the "practical theory" on which they are, and perhaps more importantly should be, practising.

Surprisingly little attention has been paid to look critically at teaching and counselling skills, their importance in the professional life of doctors and to the people they shall serve, and how these can be developed. It is high time that these shortages are rectified.

4

Education in Practice: Teaching Medical Teachers to Teach

COLIN COLES

Introduction

Continuing medical education relies on people directing their own learning. However, many may not have learned to do this. Most undergraduate courses, because of the way they are taught, often lead to a deterioration in students' ways of studying (1). So newly qualified doctors may have to develop these self learning skills very rapidly.

In this chapter, the question will be addressed as to how trainee doctors can learn to educate themselves. In particular, their relationship with their teachers will be shown to be very influential. Importantly, medical teachers need to take on the role of "educational supervisor". This role will be described, and a model discussed which teaches medical teachers to teach in a learner-centred way. Practical examples will be given to show how this can be applied in both formal and informal teaching situations.

The problems of continuing medical education

Doctors in training face a number of problems at the present time (2,3,4,5). Increasing competition for appointments and promotions means they are seeking posts that provide not just sound experience but also a good education. When they go for an interview, they look at the job itself but increasingly now also consider the quality of the teaching they are likely to get from their seniors. Medical staff have increasingly heavy demands being made on them regarding their service responsibilities. There is an enormous clinical workload, much of it carried by trainees, and senior clinicians are more and more being taken away from the wards to become involved in general management of clinical services. Clinical work requires an immediate response but education is more long term, and can all too easily be deferred until service commitments have been met. Perhaps even more importantly, junior doctors are now openly expressing their disappointment at the training they are receiving. Many feel disillusioned, stressed, and unsupported (6,7). They complain at a lack of any clear idea as to what they are expected to achieve in training posts, and are distressed at the failure of their seniors to provide systematic supervision of their work. Almost totally lacking is any feedback to them on their performance (8).

The importance of the teacher/learner relationship

While continuing medical education should essentially be self directed, the role of senior doctors as teachers remains important. Certainly, they should provide appropriate models for doctors in training grades for whom they are responsible to emulate but this implies a rather passive relationship. Effective learning, under these circumstances, is largely a matter of chance. But the authoritarian teacher is also inappropriate. This can stultify the development of the trainees or make them reliant on the teacher for their learning. Spoon feeding leads to the expectation of being spoon fed. A more appropriate model is for the teacher to be the facilitator of learning (9). Such a teacher helps the learner learn, and enables the learner to engage in self learning (10).

In the United Kingdom, general practice trainees have for many years received high quality training by being attached to trainers who must themselves have received some approved educational training. The situation for hospital training has until now been far less structured. Trainee doctors are attached to clinical "firms" led by a senior clinician or consultant, who, while being clinically sound, might or might not be a competent educator. The General Medical Council has now recommended that each trainee doctor should be attached to a nominated educational supervisor who would ensure that the trainee's educational needs are met (11,12).

The role of the educational supervisor

The role of the educational supervisor is as yet unclear, and has certainly not been fully defined. Nevertheless there are a number of situations where supervisors could provide high quality education to their trainees.

1. On-the-job teaching

Teaching should occur naturally in the course of routine clinical work. Imagine, for instance, that the trainee has been "on take" and in residence. Emergency cases have been admitted. The trainee's educational supervisor arrives and naturally wants to know what has happened, which patients have been admitted, and what particular cases, especially the difficult ones, require attention. Clearly this situation has important service implications. The supervisor needs to know how things are going, if everything is alright, and what he or she needs to be doing, and must quickly sort out what is routine and what is out of the ordinary, what can be dealt with as a matter of course and what needs particular and possibly speedy attention.

Naturally enough, the service needs must be dealt with satisfactorily. Patients are paramount. But the educational needs of the trainee are important too. Did he or she do the right things? If so, can these be confirmed? Did the trainee do something wrong, or not do something that should have been done? Does this imply faulty judgement, or some deficit in his or her competence? Was the problem the trainee's knowledge, skills or attitudes, or all three? What might the trainee do in order to cope better next time? All these are educational considerations, and the manner in which the situation is dealt with by the supervisor can, or might not, contribute towards the trainee's education. So how can the supervisor best handle these routine clinical situations in a way that helps the trainee recognise his or her own strengths and weaknesses, and know how to fill any educational gaps that are exposed, and at the same time get the service work completed too?

2. Regular educational supervision

In addition to on-the-job supervision, trainees should be receiving regular and frequent off-the-job educational supervision. This could occur in the educational supervisor's office and at a scheduled time, perhaps weekly. As with informal teaching, there is a danger that these meetings could be dominated by discussions about clinical matters, and avoid the educational implications of the trainee's work. Clearly, too, there is the danger that the educational supervisor will see these times as an opportunity to tell the trainee what he or she should and shouldn't be doing. At worst the supervisor could be entirely negative and even humiliating. Very importantly, the discussion should proceed constructively. Trainees need unambiguous feedback but they need motivation to learn too. There is the added danger that the supervisor could lecture the trainee on what he or she should know.

Clearly the supervisor has a responsibility for ensuring that the clinical work is being carried out appropriately, but so too there is a responsibility for ensuring that the trainee's education is proceeding satisfactorily. Perhaps most importantly, regular supervision should provide an opportunity for the trainee to develop the skills of self assessment. The educational supervisor has to conduct these supervisions in such a way that the trainee sees more clearly for him or herself the strengths as well as the weaknesses of his or her work, and through this sees what needs to be done to achieve or continue to provide a high quality clinical service.

3. Routine appraisal

From time to time, educational supervisors should carry out routine appraisals of their trainee's progress. Unlike regular supervisions, these appraisals would occur say every two months, and might follow a more structured approach. Indeed, the trainee's attachment could begin with an initial appraisal at which the educational supervisor would negotiate with the trainee the learning objectives of the next few weeks. Then, at regular intervals, they could review these, and set new ones.

Rather than dealing with day-to-day educational progress, these appraisals would look at the trainee's longer term goals both educationally and in terms of career progress. While the essence of an appraisal may be to assess the trainee's performance, it would also provide an opportunity for the trainee to appraise the education provided by the supervisor. An appraisal would almost certainly involve keeping records of what occurred, and of the plans they agreed together.

4. Counselling

Educational supervisors can also help their trainees through informal counselling, that is by enabling them to cope well with their work and by ensuring they have an environment which is conducive to learning. Maslow has suggested (13) that higher order mental activities, such as learning, are unlikely to occur unless basic physiological, personal, and social needs are first met. Doctors in training grades often rotate between posts gaining a variety of experiences. This is understandable and desirable but it has human consequences with little time to settle and establish good working relationships. Trainees at this time may even be establishing new domestic arrangements, and this too can be unsettling, or they could be actively considering their career pattern, and perhaps revising for postgraduate examinations. The training years often come at a time of significant personal change. Many are getting married and having families. Their parents will be ageing, possibly retiring, and even experiencing poor health. In their professional work this is likely to be a time of taking on more responsibilities, possibly becoming clinically accountable for difficult patients from which they were shielded in the very junior grades. Certainly, this is when many medical people question their commitment to their chosen profession. So, the training years can be a time of great turmoil. The trainee's educational development, under the worst circumstances, is likely to take a back seat until their personal affairs are resolved, or the two will be in unresolvable conflict with stress being the likely outcome.

Trainees have, of course, their own support networks, and have one another to discuss their progress and problems, but no matter how sympathetic one's colleagues they too have to cope with their own difficulties. Trainees can, of course, seek support in their own personal relationships, perhaps with their spouse, but this can put a strain on these too. The educational supervisor is well placed to give encouragement and support at this time, and to provide personal and professional welfare.

5. Lectures

A further role for educational supervisors is in giving lectures to groups of trainees. Lectures have their attractions. Important information can be presented to a large number of learners. It is a low cost teaching method. However, the effectiveness of lectures is open to question. They can easily foster passive learning, and even limit the scope of what is learnt. Nevertheless they are the mainstay of much medical education, and educational supervisors often find themselves called upon to lecture. Rather than doing away with lectures, perhaps it would be more sensible to find ways in which lectures could be educationally more satisfactory. So medical teachers must learn how best to do this.

6. Small group teaching

On many occasions, medical teachers are asked to give lectures to small groups of trainees, sometimes to as many as twenty or thirty, but often to as few as five or six. The lecture method is quite inappropriate here. The costs per trainee of teaching groups of this size are much greater than teaching larger groups. Small group teaching is indicated. The problem is that many medical teachers have never acquired the skills of teaching in this very effective way, and fail to capitalise on the learning that can occur.

Educating educational supervisors

If educational supervisors are expected to adopt these roles, many will quite clearly need help and guidance to carry them out. Few medical teachers have been trained to teach, and the problem is exacerbated by the fact that many of them teach as they themselves were taught. Frequently that meant sitting through interminable lectures where they were told everything they should know, and then learning facts parrot fashion to pass the next examination. Clinical competence was gained by watching others perform, and sometimes by being made to feel humiliated by failing to regurgitate some obscure fact on demand or not performing well enough at something they had never been taught adequately to do. Far from openly admitting the gaps in their knowledge, they would often hide their inadequacies behind a "cloak of competenceab" (14).

How then might supervisors be taught to carry out a more enlightened educational role? Educationists suggest that people learn best when they are helped to reflect on their own actions, identify their strengths and weaknesses, define their own learning objectives, be provided with resources and opportunities to meet these, and be able to evaluate the consequences of their learning. The educational supervisor's role with trainees would be to provide the circumstances under which this can happen, and to give support to their trainees to help them achieve it. Rather than being teachers who tell their trainees what to do and criticise them when they don't, they should be facilitating their trainees' learning by helping them to educate themselves.

In educational parlance the education that supervisors give their trainees should be "learner centred" rather than "teacher centred". This means getting trainees to look at their own clinical practice and to reflect on it, to identify its strengths and weaknesses, and by doing so to see for themselves the gaps that need filling. Their supervisors should "enable" this to happen by the way they interact with their trainees. Once trainees have seen what should be learnt, supervisors should make sure the necessary learning resources are available for the trainees to engage in self learning. While this is happening supervisors should intervene to help trainees consolidate what is being learnt, and to correct any misunderstandings or inaccuracies. Above all supervisors are there to motivate trainees to engage in self learning, that is to *want* to know what they *need* to know.

In just the same way, educational supervisors can learn how to do this. Their own educational training can be learner centred, though this time they are the learners. In practice, they can be helped to see their own educational role more clearly by reflecting on what they are currently doing educationally, to learn from this, and to change where necessary.

Teaching medical teachers in Wessex

A good example of where this is happening is in the Wessex Region of the United Kingdom where an initiative is currently underway to teach hospital doctors how to teach which draws on many years' experience of training trainers in general practice.

General practitioner trainers receive a five-day residential educational workshop. Participants bring along a video recording of recent consultations with patients. Then, in small groups together with an experienced group leader, they learn how to teach each other about general practice. The procedure they adopt has been carefully planned. Initially, two of the group engage in a piece of teaching in the following way. One of the pair shows his or her consultation video, following which the other carries out some teaching on it while the remainder of the group silently observe. Then the group discusses the teaching they observed (rather than the consultation) and they do so by using the protocol shown in Table 1.

With the group leader facilitating discussion, the person who carried out the teaching identifies what he or she believes went well in it. The remainder of the group also say what they thought went well, and the person who acted as the teacher makes a record on a flip chart of the points raised. The group leader then asks the person who did the teaching to identify the weaknesses in what happened, and these points too are written by that person on the flip chart. Follow-

Table 1.   Protocol for reflecting on practice

Begin with someone (the presenter) presenting to others some aspect of his or her practice

1. What went well, and what was the presenter's contribution to this? (Presenter first).	2. What didn't go well, and what was the presenter's contribution to this? (Presenter first).
3. What does the presenter see as his or her wants?	4. What do others see as the presenter's needs?
5. Negotiate these wants and needs, and prioritise them.	6. List the agreed learning objectives, and deal with them.
7. The presenter articulates what he or she has learnt.	8. Others say what they think the presenter should have learnt.

ing this, the remainder of the group identify the weaknesses in the teaching they observed.

On the basis of what has been said and written up, the person acting as the teacher says what he or she *wants* to do differently next time, or want to know about, and even what he or she would want to know how to do. Again these points are listed. Following this, the remaining members of the group are asked to say what they think the teacher *needs* to do differently next time, or perhaps needs to know about in order to teach more appropriately.

Clearly these two lists, the teacher's identification of his or her educational "wants" and the corresponding list of what the group sees as the teacher's educational "needs", can understandably be quite different, and there may be a need for some negotiation to occur. Through this the teacher arrives at a set of learning objectives for the development of his or her own educational skills. These are then dealt with as far as possible by the group as a whole, after which the teacher is asked to say what he or she has learnt as a result of the process. Again, all of these points are recorded on a flip chart. Finally, the group members have the opportunity to say what they believe the teacher should have learnt about his or her teaching, and this provides an opportunity to finish on a positive note by reinforcing points made right at the outset which identified the person's strengths.

Once this process has been completed another pair will volunteer to demonstrate some teaching, again beginning with one of them showing a video of a consultation and the other then carrying out some teaching on it. Once again, too, the group will discuss the teaching they observed by using the protocol shown in Table 1.

When this procedure has been employed two or three times the group leader will ask the group to reflect on what they have been doing so far, and to say what the process has been telling them about the nature of education. These points, too, will be listed on a flip chart and displayed around the walls. Following subsequent discussions of another pair engaging in teaching, all the time using the protocol to aid the reflection process, the group's attention will be directed back to the list of educational outcomes, which would be extended or amended in the light of their growing insights.

Table 2. Educational principles derived by workshop participants

Discussions are most useful when they begin with some shared concrete experience.
The learner must be the focus of education.
The learner must be given the first say.
The learner holds the pen and writes down discussion points.
Positive points must be heard before negative ones.
The teacher is the group leader, and vice versa.
The teacher acts as a facilitator, encouraging others to contribute.
The learner's "wants" can be different from the learner's "needs".
Learning objectives emerge by negotiating wants and needs.
Learners only achieve objectives (=learn) they have had a say in setting.
Learning priorities must be set.
Learning objectives can often be dealt with by the learner alone from his or her own resources.
Knowledge emerges through the articulation of ideas.
Learning occurs when outcomes are clarified.
Assessment is best when it is facilitated self appraisal which can involve peer review.
The protocol (Table 1) sets the right conditions for learning to take place. It is positive without being collusive, challenging without being threatening,

At certain points during the five-day workshop, actual general practice trainees will be brought in so that participants can carry out teaching with them, before returning to use further videos of consultations. When trainees are involved, the teaching can focus on problems the trainees are facing in their training, or on cases they have seen at a recent consultation.

By the end of the five-day workshop, participants will have derived their own list of educational principles and attributes of competent educators. A typical list taken from a recent training workshop is shown in Table 2. Interestingly it closely reflects the aims of the workshop, and is precisely the educational "content" the organiser would hope people would have acquired as a result. Even more significantly, people have learnt this without anyone lecturing them about educational principles. It was truly "self learning".

Follow-up evaluations of participants have shown that people's attitude towards teaching shifts significantly towards a "learner centred" approach; and even their attitude to consultations becomes more "patient centred" (15). Informal feedback from participants indicates that the workshop has provided them with a unique opportunity, which very few have experienced previously in their own professional education, to develop new and exciting ways of providing high quality learner-centred education for trainees in general practice. The experience of running teaching workshops in this way for general practitioners has led to the initiation of a similar development for hospital doctors.

Education in practice

What then might the medical teacher do in practice to educate his or her trainees in this learner-centred way? How in practice would they go about applying with their trainees the principles of learner centredness they have acquired at the workshops? Earlier, when discussing the roles of an educational supervisor, some examples were given of teaching situations where medical teachers could help their trainees. These will now be reexamined and ways discussed in which the principles of learner-centred education could be applied.

1. On-the-job teaching

It was suggested earlier that on-the-job teaching should occur through everyday clinical situations, so what could the supervisor do to make these situations educationally profitable as well as clinically sound?

First the trainee could be asked to describe the situation or situations giving concern, thus providing them with something concrete to discuss. The supervisor should ask questions only for clarification at this stage, and the questions themselves should be "open" rather than "closed" ones, such as "What did you do?" rather than "Did you take a blood test?" The nature of the problem (whether clinical, educational, or both) should be left open at this stage. Then the trainee should be asked to say what he believes he has done well so far, and the supervisor should reaffirm and reinforce good practice. The trainee needs to know what he or she is doing right. After this the trainee should be asked to say what hasn't gone so well, and here the problems are likely to emerge. Next, what does the trainee want to do about things at this stage? Quite often, the trainee will say precisely what the supervisor would have said, and has not taken the decision only because of being uncertain that this was right. By asking this the supervisor is doing two things: first, evaluating the trainee's competence, and second, allowing the trainee an opportunity to articulate his own thoughts, and thereby quite probably coming to see the problem and its solution more clearly. Only then, should the supervisor say what he or she believes needs to be done. This too might merely be a reaffirmation of what the trainee has already said but it might also show that they are not in agreement or there is a gap between what the trainee wants to do and what the supervisor believes the trainee needs to do. In short, there may be the need for some negotiation concerning what should happen. This should be handled diplomatically, and out of it should come some objectives whether for attending to the clinical situation or to the trainee's educational needs.

Although the trainee's educational needs and the necessary clinical provision to meet the patient's needs go hand in hand, care should be taken to distinguish between them. Clinical action will need to be taken, and so too will educational action. The supervisor should make sure that the necessary resources are available for both to be met, and should check the trainee's understanding of what should now happen. Clearly, too, at some future point, the supervisor will need to revisit the situation, both clinically and educationally, to see what progress has been made and what the outcomes are. The immediate interaction should be concluded with some positive statements on the part of the supervisor which motivates the trainee to deal with what needs to be done clinically and educationally.

2. Regular educational supervision

Earlier it was suggested that trainees need regular educational supervision, and to develop the skills of self assessment to be able to identify their own strengths and weaknesses. To some extent this will be
helped by the way the educational supervisor conducts on-the-job
teaching just described, but there is also a need for them to meet,
away from the immediate demands of their clinical work, to discuss
progress. So how should these meetings proceed?

The supervisor and trainee should meet regularly, if possible once
a week. The timing should be agreed by both parties, and the time
available, which need be no longer than half an hour, should be clear
and adhered to. Punctuality is crucial for mutual respect.

Then, the importance should be recognised of the environment in
which these meetings occur. If in the supervisor's office, and therefore not on neutral territory, every attempt should be made to limit
the effect of the hierarchical position one has over the other. Rather
than talking across a desk, easy chairs could be used around a coffee
table, and tea or coffee could be offered. Whatever the pressures of
time on both parties, neither should give the impression that they are
eager to get away.

Next the agenda needs to be set, but whose agenda should it be?
Initially, the trainee should be encouraged to say what he or she
wants to talk about, what are his or her concerns, and what is of pressing importance at the present time. If problems arise immediately, or
if the trainee makes negative comments, the supervisor should
encourage being concrete and specific, using actual examples to talk
about. Then, as already described earlier, the trainee should say what
is positive about these situations and especially to say what he or she
has done that was appropriate, or that worked well. The supervisor
has the opportunity to reaffirm this and to encourage good working
practice. Comments such as "You did well there", or "That's abso-
lutely right" or "I would have done exactly the same" would be entirely appropriate. The trainee should also be encouraged to say what
hasn't been going well, or where the problems lie from his or her
point of view. Since this meeting should be focusing directly on educational issues rather than clinical ones, the supervisor should help
the trainee explore his or her educational gaps. Having done so, the
supervisor can then say what he or she perceives these to be. Then the
trainee can be encouraged to say what he would want to know or
know about in order to fill those gaps. Clearly, too, the supervisor
will have some perception of what the trainee needs to do, though as

already seen earlier, by getting the trainee to go first, the supervisor may merely be reaffirming what the trainee has already said. As noted previously there may be differences of viewpoint which need to be explored and negotiated until a set of learning objectives can be mutually agreed. Once this has occurred, the trainee should be helped to deal with these learning objectives, possibly by being pointed towards appropriate resources the supervisor knows about such as a textbook, a journal article, or even discussion with a colleague. Importantly, too, the trainee should be asked to say what his or her plans now are to proceed with this matter, and the supervisor can reinforce the trainee's motivation by encouraging this to happen.

So far, all of this has dealt with the trainee's agenda. The supervisor may consider that other matters need to be discussed. Now would be an appropriate time to raise them. Clearly this has to be handled delicately. The supervisor might know of some knowledge areas in which the trainee has gaps, perhaps as a result of some routine clinical contact or informal teaching in the course of their day-to-day work. The supervisor should first explore what the trainee already knows in the area, especially where he or she perceives knowledge gaps, and out of this discussion the trainee should be encouraged to identify and agree with the supervisor some educational objectives, again following the procedures just outlined.

Subsequent meetings to discuss progress could deal with "matters arising" from the previous discussions, by following up what the trainee has been pursuing in the interim, and by looking at what the learning outcomes have been. The supervisor needs to show interest in what the trainee has been able to achieve between meetings and to reinforce positive learning, while perhaps correcting any inaccuracies or misunderstandings.

3. Routine appraisal

It was suggested earlier that routine appraisal should be carried out in addition to regular supervision, which would occur at the start of the attachment and then at intervals of, say, every two months. Like supervision it should be held away from the immediate work place. The essence of appraisal is for trainees and supervisors to take a longer term view of the trainee's professional development. In addition, and perhaps even more significantly, the trainee will be learning the art of self appraisal and its necessary links with self-directed learning, and ultimately self-regulated professional working. He or she will be developing ways of looking at his or her own progress, finding out how to identify personal strengths and weaknesses, and through this to be more able to set self-learning objectives. Ultimately, the aim is for the trainee to be able to do this alone without the intervention of the supervisor.

Just as with regular educational supervision, routine appraisal should utilise the principles of learner-centred education described above. At its heart this involves supervisors and trainees agreeing on an agenda which meets what the trainees want to do and their supervisors think they need to do. Once this has happened, trainee development is likely to be largely "self directed" with the supervisors assuming largely a monitoring role, giving constructive feedback as necessary.

Naturally enough, trainees like to feel that they are being listened to, and this means supervisors actually listening to what they say to them. The development of active listening skills is perhaps the single most important attribute that supervisors can acquire. Even though their own schedule is extremely busy, supervisors should make time to hear the concerns that trainees express, and show what Rogers (9) has called unconditional positive regard towards them, even though on occasions these concerns may appear trivial or unnecessary.

Trainees need also to know how to manage their own professional work in two senses, their time, and their stress. Time management should apply to their clinical as well as their educational work. Some trainees may never have recognised that they can acquire good habits of time management. For many this has never featured in their earlier education. Managing their stress is equally important. They need to be able to cope with the sometimes heavy emotional demands made by sick and dying people and their relatives. They should recognise just how important it is to get rest and relaxation, and to develop interests outside medicine. Hobbies, recreation and sport are as important to their personal well-being as a thorough knowledge of their particular clinical specialty is for their professional development. Supervisors can reinforce the importance of all of this by taking some interest in their trainee's outside interests, and by getting to know them as individuals.

Listening skills (16) require people to use open rather than closed questions, such as "How are you getting on?" rather than "Are you getting on alright?" Trainees should be asked to describe their concerns and worries, and useful phrases here are "Tell me about it" or "Say a little more about that". The trainee's feelings and emotional responses should be explored with questions such as "How does that make you feel?", which may lead on to identifying the person's own deeper reactions to his or her work with questions such as "And how are you, in yourself?", reflecting these back to them using statements like "You sound angry" or "That seems rather good".

4. Counselling

Supervisors can also help the trainee's education through informal counselling. Very importantly, when a trainee enters a post for the first time, or comes to it from another post as part of a rotational scheme, the educational supervisor should welcome the trainee and provide some kind of induction to the unit, introducing the trainee to colleagues, explaining the way the unit works and any particular conditions and circumstances that the trainee should know about. Induction schemes such as this can help trainees settle quickly. Alongside this, supervisors should ensure that the trainee's domestic arrangements are satisfactory, and show some interest into the trainee's personal well-being as well as professional development. The two are closely interlinked.

The supervisor who in the general course of events takes the approach to learning centred education described earlier will be laying an important foundation for a constructive working relationship with the trainee. This will quickly establish the principle that their professional discussions will revolve around actual practice, and that central to the trainee's education will be his or her perception of its strengths and weaknesses. Moreover, the supervisor will signal that he or she will be giving constructive and supportive feedback even of the trainee's weaknesses, and through this dialogue will be helping the trainee identify gaps in his or her education which together they will deal with. In this way trainees will quickly recognise that in this post they will be helped to develop. Very importantly, too, trainees at this time look to their supervisor for confirmation of good practice, and perhaps some acknowledgement that even a senior clinician has been in similar situations before, and felt the same way as they do now about similar matters. In this way, trainees can come to recognise that the professional environment within which they work is a positive, supportive, and constructive one, in which people are valued and respected as individuals. However, this makes its own demands on supervisors' time, and adds to their other responsibilities and commitments. Supervisors must protect their own needs. One way is to apply appropriate time management to this situation too. If problems emerge which can not be dealt with then, this should be discussed and a further time arranged when it can. Just as important is the ability to remain positive even when there are difficult problems with trainees. There is a danger that when trainees are faced with huge problems they tend to "awfulise", that is to consider that nothing is good and everything is bleak. It is also important to remain concrete, that is to keep referring to actual situations rather than deal in generalities. The supervisor should be honest too: if you don't have the answer, don't give one, if the answer is unpalatable, try to present it in the best possible way. Be clear and unambiguous about what you think and believe. Be realistic too. Do not make impossible demands of the trainee, nor allow the trainee to make inappropriate demands of you and your time. Very importantly, be accepting of the trainee's own personality – not everybody is the same. And don't take criticism personally. Sometimes in the heat of the moment trainees may make statements which on reflection they might think differently about. Be forgiving, and non-judgemental.

Overall, the golden rule in counselling is never to give unsolicited advice, and be very careful about giving advice even when asked. In the end trainees must sort out their own lives. The best a supervisor can offer is a supportive environment within which the trainee can arrive at his or her own decisions, and to provide a relationship which is conducive to sharing problems and concerns, where there is openness, honesty, cooperation, and collaboration. In learner-centred education, it is a matter of getting others to reflect on their circumstances, to see the problem for themselves, and to work out what they should be doing to resolve it or limit its effects. Only if this doesn't seem to work, or if the problem seems of a much greater magnitude than the supervisor feels competent to handle, may outside help be needed and more formal counselling agencies approached.

5. Lecturing

How can lectures become more learner centred? At first this seems impossible yet the principles of learner centredness can be applied in lectures just as much as in one-to-one teaching. Perhaps the essence of learner centredness is that teachers and learners agree on some learning objectives and then actively pursue them together. How could this happen in a lecture?

At the very start of a lecture the lecturer might ask the class to spend a minute or two reflecting on some questions. What do they want to get from the lecture? Why have they attended? How might this lecture help solve some everyday problem? Then the lecturer could say what he or she sees the objectives of the lecture to be, and what the learners might be expected to learn from it. Following on from this objective setting, the lecturer could present some example or illustration based on some clinical case related to the trainees' present work. Subsequently when presenting information, the lecturer could refer to these examples to indicate ways in which the information being taught can apply to them. During the lecture, the lecturer could pause for the class to make notes on what has been learnt so far. This could be an opportunity for taking questions there and then. The lecturer might use "buzz" groups – where people discuss a topic in pairs, or turn round to the people behind to discuss something in a group of four. Again, questions arising from this could be taken there and then. At the end of the lecture the lecturer might take further questions, and then indicate in what ways the learners could take the information further, perhaps indicating the way this particular lecture relates to lectures that have gone before, or are running concurrently, or will come afterwards. The success of a lecture can best be determined by what the learners do as a result of it rather than what the lecturer considers he or she has covered, so the lecturer needs to address the question: What will they do now with the information they have acquired?

6. Group work

Applying the principles of learner-centred education to group work is rather easier than to lectures. Certainly there are more opportunities for teachers and learners to arrive at mutually agreed learning objectives. Just as with lectures, the teacher could ask the group what they want to get from the session, and then say what the learners need to get from it. This can be helped by asking the learners to discuss some clinically related topic based on their own experience, and from this to identify their educational gaps. The resulting discussion may require the teacher to renegotiate some of the content that he or she had prepared in advance. Learner-centred education means teachers have to be rather more flexible than perhaps they were.

One feature of small group work is that, through discussions, learners have the opportunity of "recycling" their previous knowledge in a new context. This pooling and restructuring of knowledge can be educationally highly successful. Teachers and learners can be quite surprised at the outcome. The resultant knowledge is often greater than the sum of the parts.

One variant of small group learning is a workshop approach (17). Teachers can provide some educationally appropriate task or problem at which participants work. Alternatively, participants may bring along some problem from their own clinical practice to work at in a group setting. The teacher's role here is to set up the educational situation, to monitor the progress of the learners, and to facilitate the learning that occurs.

Benefits

When supervisors conduct the education of their trainees in the ways described in this chapter there will be a number of benefits. Supervisors will have a clearer educational role than perhaps they had before. Learner-centred education should, to some extent, simplify the demands being made on them for providing supervision. Supervisors trained in this way will be reassured that the teaching they are providing is of the highest quality.

Perhaps, too, working in the way described here will allow for more productive team working because of the openness it affords. It generates within the whole unit an educational ethos in which professional practices are always "provisional", and where audit occurs quite naturally. The department would become what has been described a "learning company" that facilitates its members' development and continuously transforms itself (18).

There should, too, be direct benefits for trainees. The ideas explored here emphasise the importance of service-based education. Trainees who are currently uninspired with the education they receive are likely to find the approach much more relevant to their everyday clinical practice. Regular feedback in a supportive environment will help them identify their own learning requirements. "On-the-job" learning could also mean less need for trainees to take study leave to attend educational courses, with a corresponding reduction in locum staff to cover their absence. Moreover, when a unit gains a reputation for providing trainees with good quality education, the standard of candidates applying for vacancies is likely to rise. Improved education should also mean that trainees are likely to make better decisions out of hours when referring to their seniors for second opinions. Put another way, well educated trainees will allow their supervisors fewer, or at least more appropriate, interruptions.

A further benefit of improved education would almost certainly be more efficient and more effective clinical practice, and a better standard of patient care. This might even lead to reduced litigation. A better working atmosphere should ensure a greater sense of achievement and self-fulfilment on the supervisor's part too in knowing that the education being provided is of the highest possible standard. Learner-centred education is also more fun. Teaching which actively involves learners in their own learning and self appraisal can be much more exciting and personally rewarding than teaching which is merely criticising and telling them what they should be doing.

Reward and reappraisal of teachers

In the United Kingdom general practice trainers are rewarded through extra payment for teaching, and are regularly reappraised. Nothing like this happens yet for educational supervisors in the hospital setting. Although all medical consultants are expected to teach, and have time written into their contracts of employment and job plans, there is no additional remuneration for their teaching, nor are they appraised regarding the amount and quality of education they provide for their trainees.

The "carrot and stick" of reward and reappraisal should be introduced more widely in medical education. Good teachers should feel valued. Poor ones should be identified, receive remedial help, and if necessary should no longer be asked to act as educational supervisors. The nature of these twin motivators needs considerably more debate, but the principle should be introduced that excellence is recognised in education as in other areas of a doctor's professional work, and shortcomings dealt with in some appropriate way. The teaching of future medical practitioners is too important to be an amateur pursuit. Medical education should be as professional as medicine itself.

Conclusions

This chapter has reviewed the problems that trainee doctors have regarding their education. It has emphasised the conflicts between heavy service demands and educational provision, the absence or poor quality of the feedback trainees receive, and the lack of a regular appraisal system. It has highlighted the role played by the trainee's educational supervisor who needs some form of education regarding teaching. Details have also been given of educational workshops aimed at training general practitioners and hospital doctors, and the ways in which supervision could be translated into everyday action, emphasising in particular a learner-centred approach.

The essence of learner centredness is that teachers and learners together agree on the learner's educational objectives. This can be achieved when trainees are encouraged to reflect on their practice, to identify strengths and weaknesses in it, and as a result to identify their educational gaps. They should be helped to say what they want to learn, and only then should their supervisors say what they believe they need to learn. Teachers and learners come to educational situations with their own agendas. These need to be explicitly stated and negotiated.

Once an agreed set of learning objectives has been determined, learners can often proceed with their own self education. Their teacher's role then is to monitor their progress and to intervene merely to provide constructive feedback and to facilitate the trainee's learning.

Three main conclusions could be drawn from this. First, education should be seen as a routine part of the day-to-day experience of senior clinicians and their trainees. Second, for education to be become learner centred, there may be the need to recast the relationship between supervisors and their trainees to become a collaborative, supportive endeavour with mutual respect. Third, education between supervisors and trainees requires an appropriate "climate" where trainees are encouraged to reflect on their practice, to identify their own strengths and weaknesses, to arrive at an agreed set of learning objectives in consultation with their supervisors, and to be helped to meet these objectives.

This will have undoubted benefits for trainees, and educational supervisors too are likely to gain great satisfaction from teaching in a learner centred way. But introducing a more professional approach to education carries its own responsibilities. Educational supervisors should be rewarded for excellence but also regularly appraised and face reaccreditation as educators. Those who do not meet the required criteria should no longer be asked to provide training.

It is hoped that in this way, trainees will not only acquire the necessary knowledge, skills, and attitudes for them to carry out high quality clinical care but will also learn how to learn, so as their career develops they can go even further by themselves. Continuing medical education depends on this.

References

1. Coles CR. Differences between conventional and problem-based curricula in their students' approaches to studying. Med Educ 1985; 19: 308-9.
2. Grant J, Marsden P, King RC. Senior House Officers and their training. BMJ 1989; 299:1263-8.
3. Dowling S, Barrett S. Doctors in the making. The experience of the preregistration year. Bristol: SAUS publications, Bristol University, 1991.
4. Allen I. Doctors and their careers. London: Policy Studies Institute, 1988.
5. Hunter S. Doctors in the making: How to resolve problems in the preregistration year. BMJ 1991; 303:1415-6
6. Dudley HAF. Stress in junior doctors. 1 – Stress and support. BMJ 1990; 301: 75-6.
7. Biggs J. The preregistration years 1983-1988. Med Educ 1989; 23:526-33.
8. Royal College of Physicians Education Committee. Education and Training for Senior House Officers. London: Royal College of Physicians, 1991.
9. Rogers C. On becoming a person. London: Constable & Co Ltd, 1961.
10. Knowles MS. The Modern Practice of Adult Education. Androgogy vs Pedagogy. New York: Association Press, 1970.
11. Recommendations on Basic Medical Education. London: GMC Education Committee, 1980.
12. Recommendations on General Clinical Training. London: GMC Education Committee, 1992.
13. Maslow AH. Motivation and Personality. New York: Harper & Row, 1970.
14. Haas J, Shaffir W. Ritual evaluation of competence: the hidden curriculum of professionalisation in an innovative medical school program. Work and Occupations 1982; 9:131-54.
15. Pitts J. Change in Attitudes to Consulting and Teaching after a General Practitioner Trainer's Course, MSc Dissertation. Cardiff: University of Wales, 1991.
16. Murgatroyd DS. Counselling and Helping. London: The British Psychological Society and Methuen, 1985.
17. Woolf R. Experiential learning in workshops. In: The Open University (Eds). Running Workshops. Beckenham: Croom Helm, 1987.
18. Pedler M, Burgoyne J, Boydell T. The Learning Company: a strategy for sustainable development. London: McGraw-Hill, 1991.

5

Promoting Quality in Professional Learning through Educational Counselling

KIRSTEN HOFGAARD LYCKE

Introduction

The demands on the consultant's clinical skills, medical knowledge and interpersonal insight has increased in recent years. Norwegain specialist training has been revised to improve qualifications in these areas, and educational counselling has been introduced to enhance the trainees' professional development.

"Educational counselling" is the term used here to describe a process whereby an experienced physician assists as part of an educational process a less experienced colleague to integrate and improve the knowledge, attitudes and skills needed to be a competent consultant.

This chapter will first present current developments in Norwegain specialist training to indicate the context of educational counselling. It then takes a closer look at the counselling process and discusses comparable helping strategies such as consultation, tutoring, supervision and mentoring.

The counsellors' qualities seem to be vital for the success of this activity. A training programme for counsellors and its effects will therefore be presented. Finally, some of the problems and issues still to be resolved will be discussed.

Norwegian specialist training – some current developments

In the 1980s Norwegian specialist training was analyzed carefully and found inadequate to prepare consultants to cope with future demands. Clinical education at post-graduate level in Norway had mainly been a loosely structured on-the-job training. Much of the learning that took place was in the form of an apprenticeship, which assumed that the novice learns by observing and copying the expert. There are several shortcomings to this model as an effective way of learning. Copying someone does not always give any understanding of why a certain approach is appropriate. Any attempts to adopt other approaches are thereby restricted. Practical work on the ward is certainly the most important part of specialist training, but it is not sufficient in and by itself. Learning on the wards often takes place under stress. There is little time to discuss, and little room for debriefing after emotionally disturbing events. When patients are present, deliberations may be unsuitable.

In the last decade Norwegian hospitals have suffered severe financial cutbacks with no subsequent reduction in treatment rates. On the contrary, the public demand for quantity and quality in hospital treatment has increased. These dual pressures have given trainees and consultants less time for informal exchange of experience and insight, less time to observe and consider procedures employed by colleagues, and less time to express uncertainties and give each other emotional support. Furthermore, as a result of a needed reduction of working hours for junior doctors, the number of patient encounters are reduced. In other words, factors that have sustained and enriched the time-honoured apprenticeship model of clinical training are seriously threatened.

These developments have taken place at a time of great technical and cognitive advances in medicine. Theoretical knowledge as it is taught in medical schools and in graduate courses easily becomes outdated. On the one hand, the theoretical knowledge taught may not be relevant to the practical problems of modern medicine. On the other hand, practical advances may be hampered by the doctor's lack of insight into current theoretical knowledge.

A revised programme

In order to give a better clinical training, a more sound knowledge base and better interpersonal skills, the specialist training programme was revised. Over a five-year period efforts have been made to clarify the aims and content of each element in the programme. The effects of the programme are now to be evaluated.

The main elements of the educational programme according to the written guidelines are: clinical work (including work with next-of-kin, team members and colleagues), self-study (of handbooks, articles and other literature), seminars (ward seminars or rounds), courses (internal and external), and educational counselling.

The most innovative measure was to introduce educational coun-selling as a part of the specialist training programme for hospital doctors. Before that, trainees were counselled, but usually in a ran-dom and casual way. Consultants were neither appointed nor trained for such counselling, and they had a variable awareness of their role as a model and advisor.

In what follows we shall look at the educational counselling pro-cess and compare it with other helping strategies.

The edcuational counselling process

In Norway educational counselling is used to improve the quality of education and training for various professions. Educational coun-selling seeks to integrate the individual's theoretical knowledge, practical experiences and values in order to promote professional practice (1,2). Some illustration of the counselling process in medical specialist training will be given.

A counselling session is preceded by a statement from the trainee to the consultant on what he would like to discuss. The following is an example.

Example A
HH (43) is from Iran and has applied for political asylum in Norway. He has been referred to me because his general practi-tioner suspects a heart failure. I find little in the referral that supports the suggested diagnosis, but a number of indicators of social problems and what might be psychological reactions. Addi-tional information implies that a statement from me will be used in an attempt to renegotiate the Ministry's refusal to grant politi-cal asylum. What should I do?

In the course of the day, the response to such statements is often to suggest hastily a procedure. This solves the immediate problem, but the learning outcome for the trainee may be very limited. The regis-trar will for instance not learn why this particular procedure is re-commended or in what other cases it may be useful.

In educational counselling, however, the counsellor's concern is to guide the trainee through the process of making decisions, himself making the problem-solving process explicit and demonstrating what questions a professional should ask.

Educational counselling is not only concerned with problem solving, but also with enlarging insight and understanding. The consultant is therefore advised to have three levels of counselling in mind. As a starting point the trainee is invited to explore various *courses of action* in the clinical case under discussion. How should the interview with the patient be conducted? Which examinations are needed at this point? What further information about the patient should be obtained from other sources?

Next the consultant and the trainee will discuss the arguments for each course of action. This process involves reviewing and reflecting on the trainee's *experiential and knowledge-based reasons* for his suggested actions. Are the experiences a sufficiently sound basis for action? Does the trainee have the relevant knowledge, and to what extent is it applicable to the case?

A further step in the counselling dialogue is to deliberate on the *ethical justifications* for the various actions. Are the new tests really called for or an unnecessary expense? Will further questioning be seen by the patient as an attempt to assist him or as a demonstration of distrust? The discussion of ethics in this case may go further: Does the trainee see the referral as a medical question or as a moral dilemma of loyalty to the patient or to the immigration authorities? In other words, are the doctor's personal values in conflict with the professional code of ethics?

The reflections on experiences, knowledge and values that underly these suggested actions puts new perspective on them and may call for revision of them. If the additional tests are only justified by the trainee's wish to assist the patient secure asylum, they could be discarded.

The development of the counselling dialogue in this example corresponds to a theory of educational counselling which suggests that professionals have a "practical theory" for their practice based on their personal experience, transmitted knowledge and experiences as well as their values. The professional's practical theory is *the* strongest determining factor in his or her practice. The focus of educational counselling is therefore to increase professionals' awareness of their practical theory, to challenge and elaborate on it, and to make it susceptible to change. Long-term development of quality in professional practice depends on the development of the practitioner's "practical theory" (1,2).

According to this view educational counselling should be conducted on three levels: at the level of action, of theory- and practice-based reasons, and of ethical and political justifications. This is illustrated next page (Figure 1).

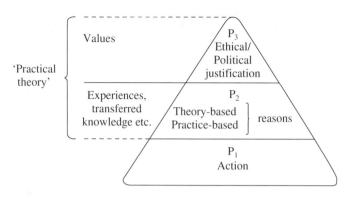

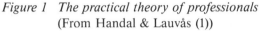

Figure 1   The practical theory of professionals
(From Handal & Lauvås (1))

As we have seen, counselling is based on the trainee's views, but he will be challenged by the consultant. Furthermore, the discussion will not be limited to one level, but rather alternate between them. For instance, when different treatments are discussed, the trainee and consultant will see them in light of the experiences and knowledge they both have as well as the how acceptable they are from an ethical point of view.

The example above focused on medical issues and the role of the physician. Educational counselling can also be concerned with the trainee's learning progress and functioning on the ward. This is shown in the next example.

Example B
As you know I have been here on the surgical ward for almost two years. My progress has been satisfactory and the tasks have increased in complexity. I used to get rather positive comments on my work from colleagues. Not so for the past months. Now I don't know what to do. Some of the patients I've treated have had postoperative complications and one had to be reoperated on. Nobody has blamed me, but I feel rather depressed. Maybe I am not suited for this – what do you think?

Colleagues often answer such statements with comments like "Don't worry – we all wonder if we should be here at times!" However, this may not reassure the trainee who may want to talk the issue over with the consultant. Again it is important for the trainee to voice his or her own aims as well as to frame the problem in his or her own way. If this establishes that surgery is a deliberate career choice, the consultant may enquire into the trainee's standards of achievement at this point and invite him or her to compare them with the expectations of colleagues. Later it may be wise to sum up the trainee's current status of experience and knowledge in the field and analyze learning needs. Has the trainee tried to go too far too quickly, or does he lack the basic skills or motivation for the work? At another level it will be important to agree on strategies to cope with the situation as it is now understood, whether the problems are due to too high expectations from senior doctors, the trainee himself, learning deficits, or something else.

It should be noted that the consultant's intention is not to control the knowledge, skills or values of the trainee, but to help him or her become more aware of them. When successful, the learning outcome of counselling is a broader range of actions to choose from, better understanding of the reasons for chosing, higher awareness of previous experiences, more self-directed learning and application of theoretical knowledge, and a deeper understanding of one's own values.

Educational counselling to some extent is ad hoc, but it is also important to plan meetings at regular intervals and to avoid interruptions. The quality of the interaction between the consultant and trainee is important, but even with regular meetings it may take some time for a good counselling relationship to develop. Therefore it might be preferable not to change cousellor when a trainee moves from one subspecialty to another, even if the consultant does not have the expert's indepth knowledge of that field. Another point is that the relationship between the consultant and trainee will change over time. The novice needs the support of an experienced practitioner, whereas the competent trainee will learn more from interaction on an equal basis.

Other guiding principles for educational counselling are:

- to make the trainee's work and situation the starting point of counselling
- to seek to extend and integrate the trainee's knowledge, skills and values
- to stimulate self-directed learning and independence
- to be emotionally supportive and intellectually challenging
- to emphasize open communication
- to evaluate the counselling over time as it unfolds.

Educational counselling and other helping strategies

The theoretical base for educational counselling is broad, but aspects of reflective practice, self directed learning and communication are easily recognized (3-9). Educational counselling in many respects resembles tutoring in that the helper will try to adopt the facilitative rather than the adviser role (10-14) and literature on tutoring therefore provides useful insights. Other related concepts are supervision and mentoring (15-16). These various strategies will be considered below.

a) Educational counselling

Counselling "... is used to denote several different activities and concerns: career advice and guidance; performance appraisal; and stress counselling" (17). Educational counselling in medicine is a process where an experienced doctor helps a less experienced colleague to integrate and improve the knowledge, attitudes and skills necessary for being a competent consultant. Counselling is part of professional education and training and seeks to relate theory and practice to enhance competent professional action.

Educational counselling covers the whole field of practice, i.e. concrete actions as well as considerations and deliberations. Reflections on practice include:

- what should be done,
- why it should be done and
- whether the practice is ethically defensible.

Counselling trainees to find their own solutions results in decisions that they will be committed to because they have personally thought the problem through and reached their own decision. At the same time trainees develop their own resources and abilities, are better equipped to manage future problems, and become more reflective practitioners.

The counsellor's aim is to increase the trainee's problem-solving capacity, without the consultant taking over the responsibility for decisions made, and without the trainee feeling compelled to adopt the consultant's understanding of the problems and their treatment. The consultant helps the trainee to perceive, understand and act upon the events that occur in the trainee's environment (10). Instead of managing the trainee's problems for him the consultant helps the trainee to gain insight into what is going on around him and teaches him how to intervene in those events in such a manner as to increase that insight and to improve the situation. These characteristics can be summed up in the following statements. Educational counselling:

- takes the trainee's knowledge, understanding, experience and values as the point of departure
- confronts the trainee's thinking and judgement with that of the consultant and the profession
- is related to the trainee's work and practical experiences,
- takes place in a one-to-one (or one-to-few) setting
- is part of professional education or training
- is conducted in conversations characterized by reflection on action and
- aims at developing the registrar's "practical theory of work".

b) Tutoring

According to Barrows (10), the tutor's function is to develop the student's thought, reflection and deliberation, sometimes called "metacognition": "... pondering, deliberating or reflecting on the problem or situation; reviewing what is known and remembered about the kind of problem confronted; creating hypotheses; making decisions about what observations, questions or probes need to be made; questioning the meaning of new information obtained from inquiry; pondering about other sources of information; reflecting on and reviewing what has been learned, what it may all mean and what needs to be done next, etc" (19).

The role of the tutor is deliberate and active. Through questions the tutor intervenes to guide the students in their thinking and stimulates them to adopt similar skills. As a result, the students naturally and automatically develop the habit of challenging each other and "deliberate, reflective, thoughtful thinking becomes a group habit through practice" (19). It is important that students acquire such skills "... as they work with life's ill-structured problems; to critique the adequacy of their knowledge and to direct their own continued learning" (19).

Barrows' ideas on the metacognitive practice of the tutor with emphasis on thought, reflection and deliberation, are very similar to what the educational counsellor does. However, Barrows' model is intended for work with undergraduate students in problem-based learning tutorials with the aim of increasing understanding of the curriculum. Furthermore, the role of values and ethical considerations on medical actions and judgements are not made explicit. Educational counselling is intended for practitioners and focuses the interrelationships between clinical practice, theoretical knowledge and personal ethics.

c) Supervision

In specialist training on the ward educational counselling can be confused with supervision. Supervision can be defined as: "... a contract-bound, time-defined, supportive, promoting and controlling process, where a more experienced colleague helps a less experienced colleague in integrating knowledge and attitudes so that the colleague improves his actions acting according to the theories and methods of his discipline" (20).

In this sense the difference between educational counselling and supervision may be academic. However, supervision usually takes place when the trainee is not yet able to perform independently according to the profesisonal standard or that the attending consultant finds it necessary to "keep an eye on him". Supervision often includes a briefing session before the event, maybe afterwards too, but the emphasis is on the accuracy of the job at hand. Advice is often directive and there is little time for reflection. More often than not the trainee will be expected to follow the strategy suggested by the consultant, not to suggest alternative procedures himself. In brief, supervision as it is practised in Norway is more directive and controlling than educational counselling.

d) Mentoring

The term mentor is used to denote an experienced professional who is a helper, teacher or adviser or even a guide, protector or source of inspiration for a junior. The relationship usually lasts for an extended period of time and is marked by emotional commitment by both parties (16).

Traditionally the mentor is not appointed but is someone the trainee seeks help from informally. The quality of the relationship is affected by personal attachment and respect as well as the duration of the relationship. The effect of the mentor on the trainee's career choice and performance as a consultant as well as on more limited daily decisions may be very strong.

In establishing a system for educational counselling, personal and lasting relationships may also occur, though this is not necessarily the case. On the other hand, the organization of educational counselling ensures that every trainee has a senior to refer to. The interpersonal quality of the relationship is very much dependent on the personalities of the two parties and cannot be forced into a particular model.

The main characteristics of educational counselling, tutoring, supervision and mentoring are summed up below (Figure 2).

	Educational counselling	Tutoring	Supervision	Mentoring
Aim	Challenge & develop theory, pract. & ethics	Learning & understanding	Control to ensure safe & efficient procedures	Maintain & develop professional relationship
Context	Postgraduate professional education	Undergraduate studies	Clinical work	Education or practice
Form	Dialogue	Dialogue	Observation, evaluation & comments	Dialogue

Figure 2   Helping strategies and their characteristics

Preparing medical doctors for counselling in specialist training

In order to prepare medical doctors for their counselling functions, the Norwegian Medical Association in 1986 initiated courses for consultants/medical specialists in educational counselling.

The courses introduce participants to theory and strategies in educational counselling and give them various opportunities to try these out on each other. In order to make the sessions realistic, participants offer examples of problems they would like to discuss with a colleague. These are usually concerned with the consultant's work on the ward. An example will illustrate this:

Example C
Our department is planning the purchase of new equipment for intensive surveillance. The equipment is temporarily installed for a trial period and I think it will be an aid to safer and more efficient treatment. I have therefore asked the nursing staff to use the equipment with an elderly woman who needs constant surveillance. The patient also has other equipment attached. The nurses react to the extra work load. The family also objects, probably because it looks uncomfortable and because one nurse has made a remark about the additional burden on the patient. What should I do now?

The participants work in groups of three. One acts as a counsellor, one as a counselee and one as an observer. The task is to enter into a counselling dialogue that adresses different levels (actions, reasons and justifications). The "counsellor" is also encouraged to be aware of different perspectives, for instance that of the patient, the nursing staff and colleagues in addition to the doctor's own perspective. Afterwards the group discusses the strategies used and the effect they had. In later plenary sessions theoretical clarification and elaboration will be offered by the course leaders in relation to problems and questions raised through the exercise. The participants' experience of such counselling exercises is that they learn more about counselling and even get help in understanding their problem better.
The major features of the course are:

Part One: Introductory Course
               (2 1/2 days)
               * Theory and strategies in counselling
               * Counselling exercises and group work
               * Lectures and materials

Part Two: Educational work on the ward
               (4–5 months)
               * Initiate educational counselling
               * Evaluate learning activities
               * Plan and develop educational activities

Part Three: Follow-up course
               (2 1/2 days)
               * Discuss and learn from experiences
               * Educational strategies
               * Follow-up on counselling

In between the introductory and follow-up courses, the participants initiate counselling with a trainee. Since counselling is dependent on the specialist training on the ward as a whole, the participants also look into this and make plans for necessary improvements in the educational programme on the ward. Reports on experiences as counsellors and on developmental work are submitted and distributed among the course participants and used as course material during the third part.

Course evaluation

By 1990, 215 out of the 8 500 medical specialists in the country had completed the training programme, covering 21 specialties and all major hospitals.

The immediate course evaluations have been very positive. Therefore the main structure and basic ideas of the course have been kept. The course content, however, has been continually revised according to feedback from participants and developments in the field.

The development of the course has been a learning experience for the course leaders as well. This has led to a further development of the theoretical base for educational counselling with improved course materials and publications as a result.

A survey study of educational counselling

Educational counselling was introduced in order to strengthen the training of future consultants. Ideas and ideals were presented but the role of the consultant and the content of the counselling sessions were open to interpretation. The courses for consultants were to promote the development of counselling theory and counselling practice.

A study of the views and practices of former course participants was initiated to enquire into what actually happens in educational counselling as well as into the effects of the courses (21). The survey study was conducted among the specialists who had completed the training programme by the end of 1990, totalling 215 persons. 190 (90%) of them responded to the questionnaire.

a) Volume of counselling activity

There is no set standard for the amount of educational counselling required with trainees in hospital specialities. Recommendations have differed from an hour each week to one hour every third month. In practice, consultants have been appointed as counsellors but never meet with their trainees for counselling sessions. An important aim for the courses has been to initiate counselling and motivate the participants to meet with their trainees at regular intervals.

The survey showed that 129 of the 190 participants who returned their questionnaire practised as counsellors. The reasons given for not practising counselling were changes in employment or their trainee had moved. Consultants not yet counselling are likely to start when a new trainee is appointed. Among those who gave no reason for not counselling are those who do not want to act as counsellors or who have tried and for some reason have been discouraged.

Sixty per cent of the active counsellors meet with their trainees for sessions at least every four weeks. Time spent on each counselling session is 30 minutes (or more) for 43 per cent of the counsellors. A further breakdown of the data shows a slight tendency towards increased frequency and length among the most recently trained counsellors.

Time for counselling is not always part of the work schedules and many counselling sessions take place outside normal working hours. In addition to planned counselling sessions, many counsellors report a fair amount of "ad hoc counselling", i.e. counselling that meets the trainee's needs, then and there. In this respect the time allocated to counselling is impressive. On the other hand, it is still an open question whether the present amount is sufficient to accomplish the goals inherent in the functions of the counsellor.

b) The role of the counsellor

The counsellors in the survey have tried out the ideas from the course in practice, and their views on their role are therefore important for future development of educational counselling. The counsellors were asked to describe different helping roles and indicate which role they would give priority (Table 1).

Counsellors emphasize the importance of helping trainees to solve their own problems and to reflect on their practice. In addition to the help given through counselling, the counsellors also find that they should be the trainee's advocate and supporter on the ward. This

Table 1   The role of the counsellor

Role	Description	% Top priority
Facilitator	Aid reflection and assist trainees in finding their own solutions	43
Advocate	Assist in practical matters and keep an eye on the trainee's well-being on the ward	40
Adviser	Support and give advice	16
Inspector	Control the trainee's work and progress	1
Total % N = 129		100

refers, for example, to cases where the trainee is overlooked when important events take place or only gets the least exciting tasks when rotations are decided. Giving advice plays a far less important role. It is noteworthy and in keeping with the ideas discussed in the course that control of the trainee's work gets a very low rating.

c) The content of educational counselling sessions

In listing the main theme of the *latest counselling session* as well as the *most common themes* we can get a fairly good picture of what actually happens in educational counselling as it is practised by former course participants. Counselling dealing with the establishment and follow up of a plan for education on the ward and further career development of the trainee is dominant. Counselling related to medical questions is also frequently mentioned, whereas focus on other aspects of doctors' work is fairly low.

This is not quite as expected. It is surprising that educational issues and not medical ones dominate. One explanation could be that medical issues are dealt with almost all the time in ad hoc counselling as an integral part of daily work. When time is set aside for counselling sessions, however, it becomes possible to talk about other issues that are not on the agenda elsewhere. With the demand for better interpersonal and leadership skills in mind, it is surprising that the functions of a doctor, in addition to the purely medical questions, receive so little attention in counselling.

Other issues in counselling are related to research and to personal matters. At university clinics there will often be research advisers who take care of most of the needs in this area. Personal matters are often avoided by educational counsellors as outside their responsibility and competence. When the actual counselling sessions are described, however, personal aspects are often the main point of interest.

This general picture of the content of educational counselling sessions does not apply equally to all specialties. Medical issues are, as expected, most commonly reported by the clinical specialties, whereas research issues are most common in the laboratory specialties. Educational and career issues are common in most specialties. Psychiatry is a surprising exception with little mention of educational and career development.

d) Course effects

Former course participants were asked to evaluate the impact of the course on their own work as educators and counsellors as well as on the educational activities on the ward. Fifty per cent of the participants in the survey (N = 190) stated that the course had been of great value. Among participants who were actively counselling (N = 129), 92 per cent stated that the course had been of great value. The participants from the first course four years ago, rated it as highly as participants from more recent courses.

As has been shown in the course description, course work is not limited to counselling. A fair amount of attention is directed toward other aspects of education on the ward. In a previous study it was shown that the course had led to significant improvements in the organization and content of the educational activities in general. It is likely that the high rating of the courses by consultants who are not acting as counsellors is due to the impact the courses have had on their general awareness of educational activities on the ward.

Not all consultants have been equally enthusiastic about the added responsibility of counselling with trainees. The discussion about these and other aspects of educational counselling, however, has created a greater interest among consultants and trainees about the general aims and activities of specialist training.

Discussion

a) Time for counselling

When educational counselling was introduced as one of the key elements in the revised training programme of Norwegian specialists, it seemed to be very difficult indeed to find time and opportunities for counselling in the work load of trainees and consultants. Several factors were not favourable; hospitals were requested to increase productivity, work schedules were tight, and counselling was not yet accepted as a part of the work schedule for the people involved.

It now seems to be a common view among consultants that counselling represents a vital addition to the other elements of the specialist training programme. However, it is certainly still not easy to find the time needed to exploit the potentials counselling represents. On the other hand, given the present circumstances, some hospitals, some departments and some individuals have demonstrated great ingenuity in finding practical arrangements that have given remarkable results in a short time. Furthermore, the attitudes on the wards toward counselling have become far more positive than they were in the beginning.

Although the amount of counselling is probably not yet sufficient to meet the aims of the project, it is still encouraging to observe the dedication of trainees and consultants to such an unfamiliar activity, inside or outside normal working hours.

b) Educational needs

The survey indicates educational needs which have become more apparent after counselling was introduced. The most apparent need is to attempt to meet on the wards the trainee's *educational* requirements. The primary responsibility of any ward is for the patients, and the educational functions can easily be overlooked unless someone is responsible for them. The fact that 40 per cent of the consultants report that their major role is to serve as the trainee's advocate is an important indicator of the trainee's need for help and support in a busy and "production-oriented" working environment.

In order to really become an advocate, it is essential for consultants to be well acquainted with the trainees and have a thorough understanding of their educational needs. Otherwise, they might easily start to direct them according to their own ideas.

c) Changing roles

Through becoming an educational counsellor the role of the consultant appears therefore to be changing from one of being the practical "helper" and "troubleshooter" to an educational role where promoting professional judgements and reflection on one's own professional work and practice are vital elements. This is an important shift. The facilitator role probably holds the greatest potential for professional development and requires the highest competencies on the part of the counsellors. Many people on the ward can help and assist the trainees in their daily work, it is therefore important that consultants now emphasize functions that are not so easily met through casual encounters.

Considering the time allotted to educational counselling, it appears to be difficult, if not impossible, for consultants to achieve their own goals and to fulfil the counsellor role adequately, especially since the time spent on counselling is often outside normal working hours. This demonstrates the unfortunate mismatch between the consultants' understanding of the counsellor role and the time available for it; unfortunate also because it is this role that carries the greatest potential for promoting professional development.

The present study shows the delicate balance sought for, and found, by the consultants between the theoretical conception of the counsellor role and the counsellor's actual functions, and how this balance is constrained by the educational needs of the trainees and the time that can be made available at present for counselling. The data alone give no indication of either the counsellor's or the trainee's frustrations originating from the mismatch of the intentions and reality, but extensive informal contacts with both parties suggest this is the case.

d) Variations in the content of counselling sessions

The survey data demonstrate a close correspondence between the counsellor's role and the content of counselling sessions. The main themes of counselling, however, vary from one specialty to the next, as do the functions of the counsellor. If we examine the reports from different groups of specialists we find interesting variations: some themes that are prominent in one specialty are absent in others. Psychiatrists often question their function in society, none of the other specialists in the sample show this kind of concern. Another example is the interest in research issues which is common in pathology, but missing in anesthetics.

It is not possible to conclude from the study whether variations as to content between specialties reflect inherent characteristics of specialties only. It is evident that counselling in a laboratory discipline must give priority to other themes than a clinical specialty like internal medicine. Psychiatry represents different kinds of challenges than orthopedics. Counsellors must transform the ideas, principles, methods and contents of counselling to match the knowledge area of the specialty in question, its procedures and methods, its patient characteristics and so on.

However, variations in what counsellors do may also reflect organisational and cultural differences between specialties. The content of a counselling session in anesthetics may differ from surgery, not only because of differences in knowledge areas, but also because of differences in organisation and tasks. Counselling in a large surgical department with a number of sections, may differ from counselling on a small ward for plastic surgery because of differences in the learning environment, attitudes towards patients, team work and/or cooperation with other members of staff.

The impact of organisational and cultural differences on what happens in counselling may add to the variations arising from differences between specialties or even subtract from them.

Conclusions

So far the development of educational counselling in medicine in Norway has proceeded as an interaction between theory and practice. We have seen that educational counselling is a valuable tool for consultants who want to promote quality in the professional development of trainees. Through the introduction of educational counselling, hospital wards have become more aware of the learning needs and potentials of their trainees. Many wards have renewed their specialist training activities and encouraged the development of the learning environment as a whole. The principles of educational counselling are based on the application of educational theory to medical practice. This perspective has proved fruitful and the course materials and publications have been well received.

The challenge now is on two levels. At one level more consultants must be made familiar with the ideas of educational counselling. The present course programme will therefore be continued. In addition, workshops for consultants will be offered at major hospitals. At another level, it is important to negotiate reasonable conditions for educational counselling, for instance by allowing consultants time for counselling as a part of their work.

Educational counselling is an innovation in Norwegian specialist training and this chapter has attempted to summarize some important aspects of the experience we have had so far with educational counselling of medical doctors in hospitals and to discuss them in a theoretical perspective.

Hopefully, the present description will instigate a debate on educational counselling as a means of improving professional quality in medical practice.

References:

1. Handal G, Lauvås P. Promoting Reflective Teaching: Supervision in Action. Milton Keynes: The Society for Research into Higher Education & Open University Press, 1987.
2. Lycke K, Handal G, Lauvås P. Medisinsk veiledningspedagogikk. Lysaker: Den norske lægeforening, 1992.
3. Cervero RM. Effective Continuing Education for Professionals. San Francisco: Jossey-Bass, 1988.
4. de Board R. Counselling People at Work. England: Gower, 1983
5. Engquist A. Om konsten att samtala. Kristianstad: Raben & Sjøgren, 1985.
6. Green JS, Grosswald SJ, Suter E, Walthall (eds). Continuing Education for the Health Professions. San Francisco: Jossey-Bass, 1984.
7. Jennett PA, Pearson TG. Educational Responses to Practice-based Learning: Recent Innovations in Medicine. San Fransisco: Jossey-Bass (in press)
8. Schein EH. Process Consultation. Volume II. Lessons for Managers and Consultants. Reading, Massachussets: Addison-Wesley, 1987.
9. Schön DA. The Reflective Practitioner. How Professionals Think in Action. USA: Basic Books, 1983.
10. Barrows HS. The Tutorial Process. Springfield, Illinois: Southern Illinois University School of Medicine, 1988.
11. Caplan G. The Theory and Practice of Mental Health Consultation. London: Tavistock, 1970.
12. Dowie J, Elstein A. Professional judgement. A Reader in Clinical Decision Making. Introduction. Cambridge: Cambridge University Press, 1988.
13. Hewson MGA'B. Reflection in clinical teaching: an analysis of reflection-on-action and its implications for staffing residents. In: Medical Teacher, Vol.13, no 3, 1991.
14. Smyth WJ (ed). Learning About Teaching Through Clinical Supervision. London: Croom Helm, 1986.
16. Yoder L. Mentoring: A concept analysis. Nurs Admin Q 1990; 15: 9-19.
17. Garrud P. Counselling needs and experience of junior hospital doctors. BMJ 1989; 300: 445-7.
18. Schein EH. Process Consultation. Volume II. Lessons for Managers and Consultants. Reading, Massachussets: Addison-Wesley, 1987.

19. Barrows, H.S. The Tutorial Process. Springfield, Illinois: Southern Illinois University School of Medicine, 1988.
20. Keiser L, Lund MA. Supervision og konsultation. Copenhagen: Munksgaard, 1986.
21. Lycke K. Veilederkvalifisering. En rapport om Den norske lægeforenings program for kvalifisering av veiledere for spesialistkandidater i institusjonshelsetjenesten. Lysaker: Den norske lægeforeining 1992.

Theme 3

Change in Medical Settings and Students as Change Agents

Knowing what ought to be done and yet being unable to accomplish change is perhaps the most agonizing experience of medical educators. In a report describing the curriculum changes taking place in a North American medical school in the fifties Williams (1) has worded the feelings of many educators faced with the challenge of change: "In the struggle for faculty receptivity... there were times when brave men of good will and high hope felt like sitting down and crying."

Change in a sense is part of the learning process and changing usually involves learning something new. The role of the educator can at times be described as that of a change agent, or change facilitator, helping the student or physician to overcome the inherent resistance to change.

Resistance to change, and resistance to learning, should not surprise anybody. Coping with both although seldom addressed in conferences or educational publications is part of being a professional educator. The papers by Gale and Grant and the one by Brattebø offer practical and very useful advice on change management that are applicable to the situations medical educators face at one time or another. Gale and Grant's paper was received with great enthusiasm by the participants at the Oslo Conference who had felt a need for just the kind of approach they offer.

The paper by Guttorm Brattebø was actually the result of a workshop at the Oslo Conference. We are indebted to Guttorm Brattebø for responding so enthusiastically to the request to write up the ideas that emerged from it for a wider audience. His paper, which is a challenge to all medical school faculties, suggests students can and should take a lead in curriculum development, and he cites situations where this has indeed happened.

---

1. Williams G. Western's Reserves experiment in medical education and its outcome. New York and Oxford: Oxford University Press, 1980.

6

Managing Change in a Medical Context

JANET GRANT*

Introduction

This paper describes the derivation and application of a model of change management in medicine that can influence change in clinical service and educational provision. The model has the unique distinction of being research-based and entirely relevant to the management of change in medicine. The model is described in detail and each of its component parts is analysed and illuminated with practical examples and illustrations. It is hoped this chapter will encourage readers to accept that change in medicine can be managed to yield better outcomes more efficiently, but, more importantly, will stimulate action through describing the steps or stages in change management in practical ways.

In late 1989 and early 1990 we undertook a major study of the way doctors liked to manage change. There had been few, if any, previous studies that had the same depth or breadth of approach. We used sound qualitative research methodology to reduce the data to a model of medical change (1,2). This model has the unique distinction of being properly based in research and being specifically tuned to the needs and culture of medicine. Other methods and models of change do exist. They are largely drawn from a distillation of experiences and sometimes lack the specific understanding of the needs of medicine. Our model was derived from the practice of medicine and has been returned to medicine in the form of two demonstration projects and numerous other minor projects. The demonstration projects are concerned with the introduction of systems for counselling and monitoring the progress of junior doctors and with the efficient management of induction processes.

---

* This chapter was written in close cooperation with Dr. Rodney Gale.

Derivation of model

We conducted semi-structured interviews with 55 medical practitioners comprising

14   GPs
11   Consultants
 8   Clinical Tutors
11   Deans and Advisors
11   Members of Statutory Bodies and Government

The interviews were based in concrete episodes of change and were tape recorded for later study. Using content analysis (3), we identified 53 separate categories that were important in understanding how doctors viewed and experienced change. Reliability studies were performed on the analysis. The most important categories are listed below and then the model of the change management process in medicine is described in detail.

An inspection of Table 1 reveals very few surprises. The most frequently cited factors are themselves a useful checklist.

Table 1. The most frequently cited factors in change management

	% of sample
1. Thorough consultation	69
2. Talking to people and explaining the changes	56
3. Teamwork	55
4. Ensuring the need for change is agreed	51
5. Ownership of the change	49
6. The use of demonstration projects	47
7. Constraints of time	47
8. Predicting potential barriers to change	47
9. The avoidance of imposed change	44
10. Awareness of timescales	44
11. Presentation of the change	44
12. Harnessing committees	42
13. Constraints of money	36
14. The personal position of the change leader	35

This list indicates our interviewees' preferred style of change and the optimal process of change. The desires for thorough consultation and for people to have changes explained to them personally mean that agreed change will be a long process. The desire for wide ownership of the change and the preference for demonstration projects also imply that slow and steady progress is preferred to untested radical changes.

A model of medical change

We used the rank order of factors to derive a model of medical change with three aspects relating to the professional characteristics and styles, the essential steps or core activities in a change programme and the tactical or style choices that must be made. These three aspects enable us to sort all the factors into a usable model of the change process in a medical context; a model that contains all the prior knowledge of change in industry and education converted to a form relevant to the special nature of medicine and the medical practice. This is because the model is derived from doctors' accounts of change. The model is a checklist and not a recipe; judgement is still needed to determine the weight of each factor in any circumstance.

Having said that the model is not a recipe, it is difficult to describe the model in a linear fashion without sounding somewhat prescriptive. Change is seldom a simple logical process where one task is completed before moving on to the next, so models give a false impression of order. We urge the reader to try to ignore the logic of the presentation which follows and to think of reality where tasks will occur in parallel and be brought up in the "wrong" order, where people will be following their own agendas. Actual change is not a logical, stepwise process.

An action plan

The remainder of this chapter is dedicated to a thorough explanation of the model of medical change shown in Table 2. This description should act as a stimulus to those contemplating or involved in change. The description of the model is itself an action plan which can be used, whatever stage your change programme has reached.

The essence of the model of change is that the bulk of the effort should be put into the preparation phase; establishing the need, ensuring sufficient power to act, designing the new system with con-

Table 2. A model of medical change

Professional Characteristics and Styles	Core Activities	Tactical Choices and Styles
Consultation	1 Establish the need	Lobbying, consultation, conjunction of circumstances, problems not solutions
Demonstration	2 Power to act	Key people, ownership, harnessing committees, authority/borrowed power, political/external power, personal position, local environment
Evolution Ownership	3 Design the innovation	Feasible? resources, timing, timescale, involvement, scale, directive/elective, degree, predicting pathways and barriers, winners and losers
Power to hinder	4 Consult	Appropriateness, leadership, teamwork, talking and explaining
Commitment	5 Publicise the change widely	Presentation, vision, amending proposals, communication
Energy and enthusiasm	6 Agree detailed plans	Detailed plans
Motives	7 Implement	Demonstration projects, scheming/bypassing, implementation, strategy opportunism, pathways and barriers to change
	8 Provide support	Resistance, overcoming difficulties, objections, maintaining change
	9 Modify plans	Compensation, modifications
	10 Evaluate outcomes	Evaluation strategy

sultation and publicity and modifying the design until it is the best that can be achieved within the constraints of time and effort available. If these aspects are properly handled, there will be far fewer difficulties when the implementation phase is reached because everyone involved will have known all about the project and will have had their views taken into account in the final design. With this careful approach, there should be fewer surprises lurking around the corner than if there is a headlong gallop to "get something done tomorrow".

We have already made clear that change is not necessarily a smooth linear process and it is quite normal to find oneself moving backwards and forwards among the various stages or processes.

Large obstacles in your chosen path may be telling you that the project, in its current form, is not viable. In which case you may wish to backtrack and find another route forward, by modifying your design or seeking new supporters. We feel that if the process of consultation, discussion and refining of ideas has been adequately carried out, then there should not be insurmountable obstacles in the chosen path.

It may happen that external circumstances change the rules of operation or the basic need for the chosen change. In these circumstances, it may be best to abandon the current initiative and try again later, with a suitably modified version.

Professional characteristics and styles

The context of medicine must be recognised and taken into account if change is to be successful and lasting. Characteristics and styles which must be considered are as follows:

Consultation. Doctors expect to be asked, to be consulted and not to be told what to do. Consultation makes good sense in that it uncovers a rich seam of ideas and thoughts. Consultation is a signalling process, it is the first step in change.

Demonstration projects. The scientific basis of medicine leads to a reliance on scientific methods in organisation too. Doctors place greater validity on the outcomes of proper trials, or demonstration projects, than they do on personal opinions.

Evolution. Gradual change is preferred to radical or gross change. An evolutionary approach allows people time to adjust to the changes and to assimilate them.

Ownership. The autonomy of doctors means that they will not generally be enthusiastic about change unless they feel they are the owners. Ownership is the perception that the changes proposed are your solution to your problems.

Power to hinder. The autonomy of doctors gives them a power of veto over many types of change.

Commitment, energy and enthusiasm and motives. Without commitment from the group leading a change, little will happen. Without the application of time and energy to the process, little will happen. If there are any suspicions concerning hidden motives or hidden agendas for change on the part of the leader or leading group, there will be little constructive progress and much bickering and resentment.

The core activities and associated tactical choices and styles

Establish the need: Lobbying, consultation, conjunction of circumstances, problems not solutions

For any proposed change, it is vital to establish the need. This must be shared by all those upon whom the change will have an impact. Perception of need is fundamental. Change is an uphill struggle, even more so without a widely accepted need.

The need may arise from a crisis, poor exam performance, student unrest, low uptake of postgraduate training, cuts in funds, for example. It could also arise in the form of the desire to effect substantial improvements in quality or reduce the effort to achieve a particular goal as a result of better methods becoming available. The need sometimes arises as an opportunity brought about by the conjunction of two or more circumstances. An example might be the retirement of a departmental head at the time when resources are available and a new Dean has arrived, or a known future reorganisation of local postgraduate education arrangements coinciding with available resources and the availability of manpower.

The hazard faced by most potential change leaders is to establish the need for change without putting forward a particular proposal to meet the need. From the standpoint of spreading ownership and gaining commitment from those affected by the change, it is essential to separate the need for change from proposed solutions. This is difficult because we often understand the need for change in terms of what we could do to improve matters, rather than in terms of exactly what the opportunities are or what is wrong. Despite the difficulty, it must be done and the change leader must promote needs, not solutions, must explain the opportunity, not his or her pet proposal.

It is also important to ensure the widest possible sharing of the need for change by consulting with peers, colleagues, Heads of Department, Deans or whoever can influence the outcome of a change initiative. The process of discussion then acts to incorporate their views and to trigger their interest and involvement. People do not like to think they have been consulted as a last resort and much prefer to be informed or consulted early in the process.

In summary, it is important to establish the need for change separate from the potential solutions or developments. Agreement on the need to do something is separate from agreement on what to do.

Power to act: Key people, ownership, harnessing committees, authority, borrowed power, political/external power, personal position, local environment

Having established a need or opportunity for change, it is necessary to look at the sources of power to move the change forward and at the forces which might hinder it.

The organisation may have the ability to change, but the change leader still needs to ensure sufficient power to carry through the changes. Power can come from positional authority or from external and political sources or from charismatic influence over others or from recognised leadership. Other sources of power arise from being a mandated representative of a group, an authority or of a Royal College. Power also resides in enthusiasm and action and it is often surprising how much influence motivated people can have.

Whatever power is to be used to smooth the path of change, it is essential to ensure that there is sufficient power available of the right type for all stages of the change process. The creative parts of the process may need a different sort of power and influence from those parts which relate to implementation and rapid problem solving. How much power and in what forms are matters for local judgement, but you do not have to use all the power you have available.

Because change has many elements of a political process, power and influence are very important. Who else is on the side of this initiative? Who is against it? The change leader who lacks sufficient personal power has several options to bring power to bear on the situation. First, influencing key people or even getting them to join in is an excellent step. Second, power can also be gained by spreading ownership of the process to a larger group of colleagues.

Another useful strategy to account for lack of personal power is to borrow some power from an important person. This may take the form of agreement to participate in the project in some limited fashion or agreement to clear lines of communication to higher authorities, for example.

In summary, power is needed to bring about change. Power can come from personal sources or from position. Power can be borrowed in the form of authority to take action or by using the good offices of a powerful person.

Design the innovation: Feasible resources, timing, timescale, scale, degree, involvement, directive/elective, predicting pathways and barriers, winners and losers

Consideration of the need for change and a review of available power will have helped to put boundaries around the possible design of a new system. Some other factors are also important.

Is the proposed change feasible? Is its scale or degree overambitious or too costly and is it within our abilities to achieve? Have we access to sufficient material and human resources to implement this proposed change? It is important to tackle something that is ambitious and worthwhile and yet remains within the available capacity. It may be wise to tackle a major change as a series of smaller ones.

The timing of change needs to be addressed. There are times when organisations suffer from what is termed initiative overload; they cannot cope with anything else.

Major changes are discussed in years and not months, the most time-consuming element being the constant round of talking to people and slowly influencing them. Given this perspective, the need for change must be an enduring one.

When a possible design is produced, it should be analysed in terms of the groups of people who are likely to be in favour of it and those who will be against it, and their reasons for this. This process, called force field analysis, can be really useful in gauging the strength and quality of possible opposition. This holds that the status quo in any organisation, at any particular time, is an equilibrium brought about by the action of forces pushing in opposite directions. There are forces promoting change and forces of resistance. The forces are ideas or opinions about the way the organisation should operate or

develop, they are the views of individuals or groups, they are sometimes inertial attitudes, they are sometimes notions arising from
society in general.

A change in an organisation necessitates a shift in the equilibrium.
It requires the forces for a particular shift in direction or behaviour
to be stronger than those who are resisting the change and trying to
preserve the current order of things.

An example of the force field for the wider use of medical audit
is given below.

Positive Forces > > > > > >	< < < < < < < Negative Forces
Improvement in quality of service and care	Another burden on time
Basis for structured edu-cational courses	Need for training
Professional collaboration	Better ways to get information
Aid to career planning	Difficult to implement
Money available, etc.	Lack of local skill
	Surgeons have their own, etc.

The astute change leader puts the maximum effort into reviewing the
forces of opposition and seeking ways in which to weaken their
effect. This may be achieved by encouraging key individuals to defect
or by changing the design of the innovation to avoid likely opposition or by incorporating opposition ideas. This review process may
show the opposition for a particular design of change to be too
powerful to continue.

A good design is one that minimises the number of people who
lose position, status or influence as a result of the change and maxi-
mises the number who stand to gain. It also takes notice of the
favourable local factors, the pathways to change, that can be a bias
to success, and the possible hurdles or difficulties that must be overcome or avoided, the barriers to change.

In summary, when designing change, it pays to look forward and
analyse the positive and negative effects of a proposal. Action can
then be taken to improve the design or to weaken the case against the
proposal.

*Consult: Appropriateness, teamwork, talking and explaining,
leadership*

When the change has been designed, it is essential to consult widely
with all those touched in any way by it, to receive feedback to help
improve the proposals and to involve those affected by the change
more closely in the events. The only limits to consultation are the
time it takes. The consultation process is a preparation for the implementation stage.

The aspect of consultation concerned with disseminating the idea
or proposal is one over which leadership can be exercised. Once
change has been put on the agenda, events may well take on a life of
their own and move in the wrong direction, unless guided by the
leadership of the individual or team managing the change. The
leadership role has to find the best balance between keeping things
moving along roughly the optimum path and taking time to consult
and discuss. Leadership demands courage and fine judgement.

There is no effective substitute for talking to people directly and
explaining to them what is going on, how they are affected and what
will happen next. It may be tempting to devise a short-cut, to seek a
way to consult with people without talking to them. Attempts to do
so by writing to them or putting up notices will cause a later backlash
of resentment.

*Publicise the change widely: Presentation, communication,
amending proposals, vision*

The consultation process is carried on with those most centrally
affected by the change, but such is the interconnected nature of the
National Health Service (NHS) and medical education that change
in any part of it can affect other parts in many ways, big and small.
The alert and concerned change leader will take every opportunity to
publicise the current state of plans and progress.

Publicity is used to alter opinions and behaviour and so the way
the changes are presented is of great significance. However radical
and innovative the design, it is always helpful to present the changes
as incremental improvements, as small changes in the previously
accepted direction.

Sometimes, publicity has to be produced before too many of the
actual details have been worked out. It is here that vision, an idea of
how things could be after the change, or an ideal to strive for, plays
a role in capturing the imaginations of others.

A large change project generates a considerable curiosity. The more people who can be encouraged to think about the proposals, the richer will be their quality and the easier their passage into existence. Feedback is valuable, but it is of diminished value unless it is used actually to amend the proposals. Listening carefully to feedback and being seen to respond positively to it help enormously in gaining acceptance.

Agree detailed plans: Detailed plans

The process of design, consultation and publicity and the impact of feedback lead to a set of proposals that are agreed and can be put into the form of a detailed plan of what is to be done, by whom and when. The change process has moved on from its free and creative phase towards its much tighter and task-orientated phase.

Implement: Demonstration projects, scheming/bypassing, pathways and barriers to change, opportunism, implementation strategy

The careful and patient preparation described so far should lead to a smooth implementation. Many change efforts fail at the implementation stage because of rushed preparation or the desire to implement the parts of a programme that have been agreed without regard for the consequences.

We have already discussed demonstration projects, or pilots, as part of the medical way of doing things, but they can also have a role in a long-term implementation strategy. It may not be possible to reach agreement with everyone concerned, but a small group may be willing to embrace fully the new methods. Such a demonstration is a way of improving proposals and of taking some of the risks away through familiarity.

A proper strategy for implementation has to be drawn up and discussed with the key players in the drama. People will have agreed why they are changing, but they also have to know what to do, with whom and when.

At the implementation stage, any residual problems or unforeseen routes to success will become apparent and active. "Pathways and barriers" is a convenient notation for all the good and bad aspects of the stages in change management and all the good and bad aspects of the choices of tactics and styles of leadership that have been adopted.

To provide a flavour of the sorts of things that were felt to be important by the participants in our study, we list a selection below:

Pathways to Change	Barriers to Change
Shock from adverse reports	Sticking to contract
Panic due to finances	Threat to status
Tradition of innovation	Protection of territory
Professional pride	Service commitments
Change of key staff	Lack of reward or gain
Supportive group	Clinical independence
Avoiding something worse	Lack of will to change
Government pressure	"Not my idea"
Incentives for acceptance	Cover-up of limitations

Provide support: Resistance, overcoming difficulties, objections, maintaining change

During the implementation stage, pragmatism and problem-solving skills come to the fore. Implementation is not the end of the process, but it is probably over halfway. People need help to assume new roles and relationships, they need support and encouragement.

There may still be some who resist the changes. Resistance amounts to qualified acceptance and is the enemy of complacency and smugness.

Sometimes when people are genuinely trying to implement change, they come across parts of the plan which do not work and cannot fit in. Such difficulties must be addressed speedily and steps must be taken to sort them out.

New methods of working are still vulnerable to regression unless the change leaders show interest and offer rewards and encouragement to those operating in the new ways. Change leaders need tact and patience to help everyone to accept and operate the new system.

One doctor we interviewed was involved in a major campaign to change the behaviour of GPs and the general public in relation to the treatment of a particular disease. This doctor found it necessary to take a new approach about every two years in order to prevent the initial enthusiasm from waning and the old ways of working from returning.

Modify plans: Compensation, modifications

Sometimes it will be necessary to redesign a system in the light of practical experience, in order to overcome difficulties or remove objections. Extensive modifications take on the character of separate changes and should be treated as such. But, do not despair, it is usually a much quicker process to modify a change in order to make it work properly than it is to start from scratch and have to convince people of the basic need.

It may be that plans are being held up by the attitudes and actions of one person or a small number of people and it may be prudent to consider some form of extra compensation, in a form available to the change leader, in order for the change to proceed and the majority to enjoy the benefits. The big danger in contemplating compensation payments, in whatever form, is that their existence is an encouragement for people to adopt extreme viewpoints and obstructive attitudes in order to be bought out and so extract extra benefits.

Evaluate outcomes: Evaluation strategy

Once the changes have had a chance to settle in, it is prudent to evaluate their effectiveness in meeting the stated purpose. This is a relatively limited, but essential, form of evaluation. It is, of course, possible to evaluate the process of change, to help with future changes and the performances of the change team members, to know what to trust them with in the future and how to improve on their performance.

It is important in evaluating the degree to which the actual changes met the perceived needs to take into account the viewpoints and feelings of the recipients of the change as well as those who led the process.

Final thoughts

Armed with a reasonable understanding of this model of change in a medical context, there should be less fear of the process. We have tried to give advice on what one actually has to do to bring about successful change. We have not told you what to change, nor what to put in its place, but we have presented a number of options for the process of change management. A much fuller account is published separately (1) containing a more detailed description of tactical choices and styles.

We would very much like to be able to provide a clear set of instructions for managing any change. Unfortunately, it cannot be done, because the best way forward depends on local conditions. It depends on the change leader's skill, enthusiasm and available energy. It depends on the local history and experience of change. It depends on the complexity of what is intended and on many other factors. The best starting point is probably to find a friend or colleague upon whom to try out your ideas, then find another and so on. The discussion process should help you to find answers to most questions and give you courage to proceed or stop.

References

1. Gale R and Grant J. Guidelines for Change in Postgraduate and Continuing Medical Education. London: British Postgraduate Medical Education, 1990.
2. Gale R and Grant J. Managing Change in a Medical Context: Guidelines for Action. London: British Postgraduate Medical Education, 1990.
3. Berelson B. Content Analysis in Communication Research. New York: Hafner, 1971.

7

Turning the Tide:
Medical Students as Change Agents

GUTTORM BRATTEBØ

Summary

Medical students could become a unique and powerful force in the evolution of medical school curricula. Unfortunately, the significance of this potential is seldom fully recognised, either by the students themselves or by their teachers. In this chapter various ways are discussed in which students can make an impact on the curriculum and the educational activities in medical schools, and some of the problems this creates are considered. The importance of increasing the students' awareness of fundamental pedagogical issues is emphasised, including their vital role in developing their own learning environment. This process should start during the first year of medical school. The chapter was the result of a productive and valuable workshop at the Oslo Conference in which both medical educators and students participated, coming from medical schools with curricula ranging from the most traditional to rather progressive ones. Because of this, the principles outlined here should apply very widely.

Introduction

Medical schools need constantly to be evaluating their curricula. Without this the evolution of medical curricula is a slow process. Recognising the fact that medicine must change in response to society's needs, the field of medical education is now expanding rapidly. Medical students are the people who most directly experience these changes, and so are well placed both to monitor their curriculum and to implement change. Students should be encouraged to play an active role in the change process, and if stimulated in the right way can become a leading force in the evolution of educationally sound curricula.

Without doubt medical students are potentially capable of influencing their educators greatly, a fact which is reflected in the saying that "one learns as long as one has students". Having said this, traditionally it is the teachers who dictate the changes that occur. Seldom are medical students invited to have any real influence on the process, because the value of their key position is not appreciated in most medical schools (1).

Sadly, often the so-called "new" curricula in "old" medical schools seem merely the equivalent of "re-arranging the deck chairs on the Titanic"! This is partly a result of not involving the medical students in the change process at a very early stage. On the contrary, the view is commonly held of medical students as passive consumers who are to be spoon fed every medical fact believed to be of relevance in a given discipline. Too much emphasis is also placed on technical aspects of the curriculum such as timetabling, rather than questioning what actually goes on. Students are great survivors too. They have been shown to develop various learning styles, which have a significant influence on their success at medical school (2,3). They have considerable insight into the education they are receiving.

So if medical students want to improve the educational value of their curriculum, what is the potential for involving them as fully as possible in curriculum change?

Features of medical students

Students entering medical schools are young, intelligent and eager people, who are capable of becoming excellent learners and physicians. They have courage, endurance and self discipline. They are capable of taking advice from their teachers, and if motivated are willing to put in enormous efforts to reach their goals. However, the people responsible for medical curricula seldom appreciate this unique opportunity, and instead of cultivating the curiosity and educational appetite of the junior students, "lecture them to death". Very soon students lose interest and the first "golden opportunity" is lost. Medical school is seen as something to survive rather than a true university education. Later the un-doing of this can be as time-consuming as it is painful.

While in some places time and effort have been spent on improving the educational skills of teachers, it is not often realised that students could also learn more about education. A small introduction to study skills and pedagogical principles could enable them to make the most of their educational experiences and so become better learners (4).

At the University of Oxford Medical School it was proposed to abolish the formal final examination, relying on what were considered the more valid and comprehensive results from a continuing assessment programme (5). However the students wanted to keep the final examination because they believed that passing such a hurdle gave them self confidence and experience for dealing with postgraduate examinations.

It is even possible to use senior students as resources for junior students, as tutors, though here too there is no tradition for this in most medical schools. Where it has been used, it seems to function very well. This was the main conclusion from a pilot project (6) at the Law School at the University of Bergen, where the failure rate dropped among the students who had participated in small groups led by senior students. As well as being introduced to sound educational principles, these groups discussed the core items from the curriculum, and this motivated the students to write assignments, take better notes, and revise fully for the final examinations.

The rules of the game

One problem for medical students who want to be involved in changing aspects of their curriculum is that they do not know the various channels, whether formal or informal, within the institutions through which it is possible to influence others. Senior students who have been living with the system for some years have acquired considerable knowledge about the channels of influence within the medical school, and the sharing of this wisdom with junior students should be encouraged. Experience of this at the medical schools in Bergen and Tromsø (7) has shown that informal contact between students has led to them organising a number of important conferences on medical education, as well as the establishment of teaching critique groups.

Lobbying is another important way of influencing change in a medical school's curriculum through the established channels such as the faculty board or curriculum committee. It is also possible to seek support from the national medical association, perhaps through contact with physicians who are interested in medical education. In Norway the medical students' association became part of the Norwegian Medical Association (NMA) in 1988 and was recognised as a special branch with nearly all the privileges of full members! National organisations of university students may even have an impact on the legislative bodies within the national health service and university authorities. These students' organisations also possess valuable organisational knowledge, and cooperation with them stimulates a change process in individual medical schools.

Strategies

The choice of strategy students adopt will depend on local factors, and to a certain degree on the resources available. One way of classifying different change strategies is to group them according to their costs and degree of faculty involvement needed. This is schematically outlined in Table 1. Low cost strategies may or may not be faculty dependent. High-cost strategies, on the other hand, are often dependent on faculty members helping students secure the necessary funding because of their wider contacts and experience in fund raising, and deeper knowledge of sources of funds and of ways funds can be obtained. Consequently, it may be advisable to start off with the low-cost and faculty independent strategies first and then turn to the more demanding ones later on.

The first step for any change is the definition of the problems in the present curriculum to be attacked. The concept of "sharing the problem" is central in this phase. This may mean students clarifying what the educational problem really is and helping faculty see this too without alienating them in the process. Ultimately, faculty have to understand the problem and share the students' sense of its

Table 1 "Student Change Strategy Table" (SCST)
A table in which the various change strategies can be grouped according to their costs in money and manpower. Depending on local factors it is wise to start out from the upper left cell.

	Faculty non-dependent	Faculty dependent
Low cost strategies		
High cost strategies		

importance. Some kind of survey of students might contribute towards this, provided the methods used meet acceptable standards of educational research. The costs need not be great as the students themselves can carry out a lot of the labour intensive work.

Some years ago a group of medical students in Bergen managed to get acceptance for doing a survey of this kind as a project in community medicine at the medical school. They published the results in an international journal for medical education, proving that medical students are capable of producing high quality research reports (8). The article has often been referred to in the debate over the Norwegian undergraduate medical education.

Table 2 lists some desirable characteristics of innovations in medical schools, based on research (9,10). Paying attention to this list

Table 2   List of desirable characteristics of innovations in medical education, modified after (10,11)

Characteristic	Means
Relative advantage	New valued benefits accrue from the new programme. Students might learn more, faculty might be more satisfied and interested in their work; more efficient time use.
Compatibility	The new programme must not conflict radically with existing value systems or codes of behaviour.
Simplicity	Although the reasons for a change may be compléx, the new program should be easy to understand and easy to participate in. False barriers of complexity should be reduced as much as possible and the system should be well explained.
Trialability	A change should be designed so that it could start on a small experimental scale, and be modified if needed.
Observability	Potential adopters or participators must see what is happening when the system is applied on a trial basis, and non-participators should be able to obtain enough information that they can convince themselves that they too should participate.

could improve the probability of acceptance by the faculty. The points on relative advantage, and trialability are particularly important to consider before presenting a change plan.

Some senior faculty members seem to think that the students' perception has a very limited value such that it cannot contribute to curriculum reform, but the students must believe that their input is important. One report on evaluation of university teaching notes: "A review of recent research concerned with student ratings of teaching indicates that such evaluations are not significantly influenced by background variables, and are valid, reliable, stable, generalizable, and useful." (11). This view is also supported by others. In his book on evaluation of teaching in medical schools, Robert M. Rippey argues that "While other sources (of evaluation data) may contribute additional insights, student evaluations must form a cornerstone of any evaluation program because of their perspective, their intimacy, and their long hours of contact with the instructional process." Only the students know the entire curriculum at a certain time. Would a senior professor be prepared to go through medical school again, or sit the final examination? (12).

There are now many reports of alternative curricula in undergraduate medical education. This resource should not be viewed as exclusive to medical educators. Medical students should draw on it too and use it in striving for the "best" curriculum. If students can refer to a scientific publication, thereby proving that it is possible to do things in another and perhaps more acceptable or better way, this will have more impact than merely negative criticism of the existing curriculum. It is very important to provide alternatives, instead of just telling the teachers how bad things are. This is after all the way physicians and researchers argue their own case in the academic medical world. It may be difficult for a teacher to turn down constructive suggestions from the students that have been well researched elsewhere.

There are also many ways dull lectures and seminars can be improved and made more interesting for the students. Booklets on this have been published (13,14,15), and it might be useful to provide teachers with a copy. Performing a diagnostic work-up of medical school courses, following the same outline as used in the diagnostic process of patients, can be an enjoyable exercise, at least for the students (16). Giving the teachers copies of scientific articles on medical education and learning is also an easy and low-cost way to influence the system (Table 1).

In academic medicine the concept of peer-review is now becoming more widely accepted as a means to quality assurance. This principle can also be applied to medical education to improve the quality of the instruction offered. For example, it might be possible to invite a teacher interested in medical education to sit in on a colleague's lecture or seminar and then to comment on the teaching (17). It can be very interesting to see the impact of this on the teacher who knows that he or she is being peer-reviewed.

Open educational meetings with panel discussions or invited speakers can also be important in the promotion of an idea. Teachers and students then both have to express and defend their ideas especially if they are well thought out and fully evaluated.

If a particular part of the curriculum has been identified as being a problem, students could form a "trial and error group". The use of small "pilot projects" can be an important step in the change process. This approach is especially of significance in the larger and more conventional schools, which tend to be prestigious and less likely to accept large-scale innovative change all at once. Sometimes it is possible to get funds for such small-scale trials. If the project turns out well the medical school programme can be expanded. Projects in which those who are keen and interested work together can act as a catalyst for further change.

Sometimes where there is a great indifference amongst teachers to curriculum change, it might be considered acceptable to take the calculated risk of direct confrontation but such a strategy must be taken only with great caution! At the Karolinska Institute in Stockholm a small group of students once occupied the podium and grabbed the microphone from an anatomy teacher, demanding something be done with the course which had been criticised by students for years without any response from the faculty. This somewhat drastic action did in fact have a major impact both on the teacher and the other students, and the course did change. However, as a strategy for change it is not to be recommended everywhere!

Problems

The students' understandable ignorance of educational principles and alternatives has already been mentioned as an impediment to the change process. While this can be overcome, however, there are other factors which are harder to be accommodated. One obvious problem is the fact that medical students are short lived. They spend only five or six years at medical school, where at least the first and last years are likely to be unproductive as far as curriculum development is concerned due to unfamiliarity with the system and lack of time. Now and then individuals make a great impact on the system but suddenly they are gone and things can return to normal. Better contact between the classes would help.

At the same time, though, the ever changing student body can provide refreshing and unprejudiced attitudes. Perhaps this can turn an apparent weakness into a strength for curriculum change.

Another impediment can be the individualist who creates bad student-teacher relationships, and even strengthens the authoritarian climate so that criticism is not accepted. Unfortunately, such an extreme climate will eventually foster anger amongst students who might then take some drastic, and probably counterproductive action. One way of dealing with this would be for the medical school to introduce a system of greater feedback between students and teachers (18).

There are now several instruments (19) which can be used to measure the educational climate of a medical school. No dean would like to see that his own medical school scored badly on such an inventory, and therefore studies like this could be a useful start, showing that there is something to improve. Of course, even when students have criticised the curriculum or collected data to support their view, the faculty might still not take the students seriously, or simply state that the suggestions being made are impossible to adopt. Such resistance must not be accepted. The more coherent and responsible the students are, the more they can demand changes to the system. Some students may face becoming unpopular with faculty members who are upset by the idea of change, and even feel this could affect their progress. If these threats are based on reality, clearly there is a serious problem that needs dealing with at a high level.

Conclusions

Medical students are a valuable resource which should be far better utilised in the pursuit of improvements in their undergraduate education. To do so they should become familiar early on with the fundamental principles of human learning and the educational alternatives that already exist. Educators and senior students should share their knowledge with junior students. Enhanced contact between students and faculty will help the change process, and also enable students to take a responsible approach in helping with curriculum development. In particular, students must share with faculty the educational problems they are experiencing, possibly through carrying out a survey as widely as possible in their medical school.

The discussion in this paper is not meant to be exhaustive or complete but a brief introduction to this fascinating way of approaching changes in medical schools. If just a couple of medical students take up some of the ideas brought forward here, the primary goal for writing this chapter will have been reached.

Acknowledgement

I would like to thank Dick Mårtenson for fruitful discussions and for his helpful suggestions in the preparation of this chapter.

References

1. Centra J. Effectiveness of student feedback in modifying college instruction. J Educ Psychol 1973; 65: 395-401.
2. Coles CR. Differences between conventional and problem-based curricula in their students' approaches to studying. Med Educ 1985; 19: 308-9.
3. Mårtenson DF. Students' approaches to studying in four medical schools. Med Educ 1986; 20: 532-4.
4. Mårtenson D, Brattebø G. An introductory pedagogical survival course for first year medical students: a brief account of the course. Med Educ 1992; 26; 340-2.
5. Weatherall DJ. Examining undergraduate examinations. Lancet 1991; 2: 37-9.
6. Skjold-Wilhelmsen L. Evaluering av "Jus-prosjektet" ved Universitetet i Bergen. Det juridiske fakultet, Universitetet i Bergen, 1990.
7. Endresen PC, Brattebø G. Pedagogisk eksperiment: "Survivalkurs" for Tromsøstudenter. Tidsskr Nor Laegeforen 1991; 111: 2305-6.
8. Kaisen A, Kjetså GA, Lie RK et al. Interns' evaluation of their preparation for general practice: a comparison between the University of Tromso and the University of Bergen. Med Educ 1984; 18: 349-54.
9. Carpenter-Haffman P, Hall G, Sumner G. Change in education. Cambridge: Ballinger Publishing Co., 1975.
10. Rippey RM. The evaluation of teaching in medical schools. New York: Springer Publishing Co., 1981.
11. Overall JV, Marsh MH. Students' evaluations of teaching: an update. AAHE Bulletin 35, 1982.
12. Evans MJ. Sacrificed to an archaic training system. BMJ 1991; 303: 65.
13. Gibbs G, Habeshaw S, Habeshaw T. 53 interesting things to do in your lectures. Technical & Educational Services Ltd, Bristol: 1984.
14. Habeshaw S, Habeshaw T, Gibbs G. 53 interesting things to do in your seminars and tutorials. Bristol: Technical & Educational Services Ltd, 1984.
15. Habeshaw T, Habeshaw S, Gibbs G. 53 interesting ways of helping your students to study. Bristol: Technical & Educational Services Ltd, 1987.

16. Whitman NA, Cockayne TW. Evaluating medical school courses: a user-centered handbook, Utah: University of Utah School of Medicine, 1984.
17. O'Byrne GA. Are doctors born teachers? BMJ 1988; 296: 838-9.
18. Ende J. Feedback in clinical medical education. JAMA 1983; 250: 777-81.
19. Fraser BJ, Treagust DF, Dennis N C. Development of an instrument for assessing classroom psychosocial environment at universities and colleges. Studies High Educ 1986; 11: 43-54.

Theme 4

The Technology of Teaching and Learning

This theme brings together two quite different chapters. The first, Chapter 8, looks in depth at the importance of new technology in the development of medical education, particularly as it affects general practice. The author suggests that new technology is providing doctors with a source of considerable knowledge to help patient management directly in the clinical situation. One clear implication is that doctors will no longer need to carry in their heads so much diagnostic information as they do now. Rather, during consultations, they will have the opportunity to concentrate on the communication process itself, and the patient's social, psychological, and emotional state. A second implication is that doctors will not need regular updating of knowledge as this will happen automatically through their computers. Routine updating will focus more on developing their professional practice and auditing its effectiveness. All of this has implications for medical education which will need to be very different from what it is now.

Chapter 9 reminds us of the vital role still to be played by what might be called the "old technology" of medical education, that is of reading and writing. Whatever developments occur in information technology, these will remain central features of medical education. They provide not just the tools for self learning but can contribute greatly to extending the learner's horizons. The chapter stresses that for education to be effective, the learner must be actively engaged in the learning process, and literature is an important resource for this process. Very important, too, is the enormous range of literature available to people studying medicine, and this should be utilised as effectively as possible in broadening the doctor's mind aesthetically. Medical education should be concerned not just with knowledge acquisition but with the development of appropriate attitudes and values. The chapter concludes by briefly discussing how to write better, and provides important insights into what is needed in order to communicate effectively.

On their own, both chapters make an important contribution. Taken together they are provocative and full of insight.

8

Learning, Knowledge and New Information Technology: Present Issues and Future Prospects

PETER PRITCHARD

1. Introduction

Medical information technology has now developed to a stage when we have to question its likely impact on learning in general and on medical knowledge transfer in particular. Knowledge-based systems (KBS) that are now being developed for general practice could radically alter the way general practitioners work, and could provide them with a very large distributed knowledge base, as well as supporting decision making in the consultation. KBS could also foster evaluation and learning with the powerful tool of "concurrent audit", linking the decision process to patient outcomes, with a profound impact on the quality of medical care. By making the referral process more logical and effective, the balance between primary health care and the more costly secondary and tertiary care would need to be reassessed.

The technical benefits that might accrue to patients and doctors must be balanced against the risk of the consultation becoming more technical and less empathic. Furthermore, there might be less attention to "knowing-in-action" and "reflection-in-action" as the essence of professional learning and practice.

Postgraduate education of general practitioners might need to focus more on communication and decision-making skills, and less on the acquisition of volatile biomedical knowledge, with more use of in-house and small group learning.

Historically, the adverse social side-effects of new technology have been learned too late. Perhaps, on this occasion, educational measures can be in place in anticipation of the technology.

The private consultation between patient and personal physician (or other health professional) is the idealized focus of health care in the

United Kingdom. In such a consultation, rapport and empathy are established; knowledge is exchanged; skills both technical and interpersonal are employed; and mutual attitudes and beliefs explored. That is not how it always works out, but it represents the sort of model to which professionals (1) and patients aspire (2).

Doctors have traditionally tended to concentrate on biomedical knowledge and on ways of transferring their knowledge to the patient. Early in the present century, general practitioners tended to keep their knowledge to themselves as a precious commodity on which their livelihood depended.[1] The patient's story was often elicited in response to closed questions (3) rather than a mutual exploration of biographical events and their interpretation.

Michael Balint (4) profoundly influenced British general practitioners away from the notion of diagnosis and treatment being an impersonal ritual and towards a more transactional view of the consultation, in which the doctor's personality was a key factor in helping the patient and doctor to learn from each other. More recently, the importance of communication skills has been demonstrated scientifically with the work of David Pendleton and colleagues (5) and Philip Ley (6). The patient's health beliefs may determine whether medical advice is accepted or rejected more precisely, a mismatch between the patient's and the doctor's beliefs and the working models of health and sickness to which they relate their daily experiences. The nature of these beliefs and models can only be discovered by enquiry, and this line has not been pursued very actively in medical education, though some medical schools do have a formal structure for patients to act as teachers.

Doctors may find it hard to admit that the medical model has its limitations and that the patients' knowledge about themselves and their view of the world is important. The concept of communication on the basis of equality between adults has a long history (8), yet the doctor-patient relationship, by maintaining the traditional "parent-child" interaction, inhibits the two-way flow of knowledge. David Tuckett and colleagues (9) characterized the consultation as a "meeting between experts" and stressed the importance of sharing ideas.

---

1 The GP father of Dr William Pickles, the first President of the Royal College of General Practitioners, is quoted: "If patients ask me what is the matter with them, I tell them 'that is my business – just take the medicine and you will get better'".

This recognition of the importance of the patient's knowledge must be taken into account when considering the entry of a third participant, namely the knowledge-based computer system,[2] into the transaction. Indeed, the general public has access to many sources of biomedical knowledge, through the media and through self-help groups, in a detail that hardly existed ten years ago. General practitioners are now expected to cover a wider spectrum of knowledge including the social dimension. But all the time the quantity and complexity of biomedical knowledge is increasing at such a rate that the generalist is bound to be overwhelmed (10). Specialties in medicine fragment into sub- and super-specialties, and more non-medical and non-nursing experts are included in care teams. Thus the knowledge gap between general practitioner and specialist widens to the point that communication becomes less effective, and mutual confidence is lost. Similarly, the patient may be disappointed in the general practitioner as a fount of accurate and up-to-date knowledge, and as a guide through the complex pathways of secondary and tertiary medical care.

Conventional computer systems are becoming the norm for UK general practice, and over 90 % of practices now use them. Increasingly they are being used for patient records, available on-screen in the consulting room. It is only a small step for medical knowledge in text form to be available to the doctor during the consultation. Several systems exist to do this. An important step would be for approved treatment guidelines to be available on-screen, to help the GP to conform to accepted practice and to avoid mistakes (for example in prescribing). Simple systems to support decision making already exist, but are fallible.

More robust systems await the full development of knowledge-based decision support systems such as the "Oxford System of Medicine" (11,12). Such systems should be able to make relevant information available to the doctor at the appropriate time in the decision-making process. This could be knowledge of whose existence the doctor was unaware, or had long forgotten. Knowledge-based systems have great potential for improving the effectiveness of care

---

2 These computer systems are sometimes referred to as "expert systems" employing "artificial intelligence", or 'fifth generation' computer systems. The author prefers to avoid these misleading terms, and stick to the term in the main text. 'Knowledge' in this context refers to "knowledge with which to perform reasoning" (Oxford Dictionary of Computing 2nd edition).

in general practice, and for rationalizing the process of referral to hospital (13). However there are a number of caveats.

First and foremost is the point that making effective decisions in general practice must depend primarily on what Schön (14) has called "knowing-in-action", which, as he stressed, is not the same as knowledge gained in college or from textbooks, but rather an accumulation of case experience (see section 2). To develop the level of knowing-in-action requires "reflection-in-action". Will new information systems encourage reflection-in-action or inhibit it? Furthermore, will they encourage an exploration of patients' knowledge and health beliefs or the reverse? Will the new-age computer become a useful tool, or will it enslave the doctor in its rituals? These issues are discussed in later sections.

Presenting the general practitioner with knowledge at the precise moment of need is very different from current educational practice, which depends very much on pre-knowledge, or looking-up after the event. Seeking knowledge during the consultation is often inhibited by cultural taboos (15), and by the inability of existing information systems to provide instant, relevant and clutter-free information. The content and the balance between essential pre-knowledge and look-up knowledge might be radically altered by knowledge-based systems. In addition, there is the potential for the system to take the initiative by supplying new knowledge during the consultation in the form of prompts, like a critiquing colleague or an automatic textbook. Current postgraduate education, ineffective as it may be (16), may be able to change its focus from communication of knowledge (e.g. recent advances) to skill training and enhancing reflection- and knowing-in-action.

The lesson of history is that technological advance has a momentum of its own, and has serious social side effects which are rarely predicted nor mitigated. We do not seem to learn from past errors (17). So the costs of a fundamental change such as the use of knowledge-based decision support would have to be balanced against the benefits. That is difficult to do without hindsight, but the challenge to teachers and learners of medicine is inescapable.

This introduction has raised a number of issues, and these will be addressed in subsequent sections as under:

- What is the present state of biomedical knowledge and what kinds of knowledge are appropriate for knowledge-based systems? (Section 2).

- What is the current state of development of knowledge-based systems (KBS) for general practice? (Section 3).
- Can the effectiveness of the process of referral of patients to hospital be improved by knowledge-based systems? (Section 4).
- What impact might KBS have on professional learning and education, particularly as regards communication of knowledge? (Section 5).
- What impact might KBS have on patients' knowledge and on communication in the consultation? (Section 6).
- What future prospects are likely, and what is the balance of costs and benefits of implementing advanced information technology? (Section 7).

2. What is the present state of biomedical knowledge and what kinds of knowledge are appropriate for knowledge-based systems (KBS)?

Biomedical knowledge is expanding at an exponential rate, and the response of hospital specialists and researchers is to split into more specialties. By contrast, the general practitioner in UK and many other countries, has tried to remain a generalist, and retain enough knowledge of each specialty to carry out everyday tasks, and to know when to refer to a specialist and if so, to which specialist. In addition to the fragmentation of biomedical knowledge, the general practitioner, as already mentioned, is expected to extend the range of knowledge into psycho-social areas where the level of certainty is even less than in biomedicine. It is no wonder that the general practitioner feels under pressure, and their ability to cope is called into question. Yet as specialist medicine expands, so does its cost, to the point that no country can afford a fully comprehensive health service (18). As a consequence, the generalist's role as a referral agent and gatekeeper becomes all the more important. This is reinforced by the WHO/UNICEF (1978) Declaration (19) which stressed the role of a revitalized, community-oriented primary health care service. Accordingly, the knowledge needs of primary care need to be addressed and their functionality assessed.

The general practitioner has an ever wider knowledge gap to bridge. To what extent could this be helped by knowledge-based systems? We can expect them to exert a favourable influence on the GP–specialist boundary: whether they can have an impact on the patient–GP boun-dary remains to be seen. But first let us look at the state of knowledge production and utilization in biomedicine as a whole.

The information avalanche

Medicine as a whole is pushing out its frontiers at an alarming rate. Biomedical information is becoming more plentiful, complex and fragmented, and each fragment occupies a narrower domain which is now shared with many more non-medical scientists. This fragmentation of specialties is an inevitable and expensive consequence of progress, but as a result, general practitioners are now the only generalists in medicine and the quantity and range of information which they need to handle continues to grow. If they can only just cope now it is unlikely that they will be able to do so in five or ten years time (10).

The flood of new publications presents serious problems for the medical community since relevant information is scattered throughout many journals and books. According to Weiss (20), 8–10 million scientific and technical documents are now published annually, among them 75,000 books and 300,000 patents; and 6–7 thousand scientific articles are written each day. 54,496 articles on oncology have appeared in 1,038 journals between 1969 and 1974 (21). Moreover, one study estimated that 70–80 % of all publications are without any practical importance and Weiss (20) calculated that about 50 % of published literature is never used. A study at the British Library of Science and Technology, cited by Weiss, showed that, in a one year period, 4,800 medical journals out of 9,120 were not consulted; 80 % of loan requests were filled from 900 titles and 50 % from 40 titles.

The "knowledge production system" may be able to justify some waste products, but the current user, when faced with this mountain of paper knowledge, has difficulty in deciding what knowledge might be useful. Useless knowledge is not discarded. It just clutters up the system until time and cost dictate a wholesale discard of the good and the bad. Viewing knowledge as an open system, the inevitable conclusion is that there is overproduction of knowledge of dubious quality and under-utilization of the potentially useful knowledge, due to lack of a discriminatory feedback mechanism to maintain the stability of the system.

General practitioners now need to handle an increasing quantity and range of medical information, but the difficulty of selecting important information from the mass of publications is a particular problem for them, since their required knowledge has to cover so wide an area. In order to keep up with pertinent scientific developments, GPs find themselves swamped with information that they have little time to assimilate or even to scan. Numerous studies have shown that important new findings reach this professional group rather late or not at all. A project undertaken in Germany found that 40 % of the physician sample did not know any contraindications to oral contraceptive agents, 30 % knew one and 20 % knew two (22). Another study (23) found that only 38 out of 137 family physicians (28 %) were aware of the results of a trial of photocoagulation in diabetic retinopathy published eighteen months previously, and only 33 % who were asked to handle two patients' problems (related to diabetic retinopathy) did so correctly.

Weiss (op cit), in an analysis of the users of biomedical information, suggested that general practitioners have little time or motivation to read. This view confirmed that of Dr Annis Gillie, former president of the Royal College of General Practitioners who wrote "the full educational scope and its demands that face us today has little reality for many among the mature and often very weary doctors in practice" (24). Sir William Osler said it more bluntly early in the century with his aphorism: "It is astonishing with how little reading a doctor can practice medicine, but it is not astonishing how badly he may do it".

Current library and information systems do not provide the instant kind of information that GPs need in the consultation. They require answers to clinical problems quickly and reliably and they want readable and comprehensible information in language that they (and their patients) find easy to grasp. Barley (25) suggested further reasons why GPs rely more on their wits than written sources. First, they practise rapidly and in such a way that the patient, by repeated visits, provides the answer. Secondly, if they do not know something then they can refer to someone who does, so there is no premium on finding out for oneself. Finally the field of work is so vast that it is often tempting to decide to keep a good working knowledge at one's fingertips rather than become an expert in matters of detail.

Disease, illness and the biomedical model

"Disease" refers to a medical conception of pathological abnormality which is indicated by a set of signs and symptoms. "Illness" on the other hand, refers primarily to a person's subjective experience of "ill-health" and is indicated by the person's subjective feelings of pain, discomfort, etc. (26). Modern physicians are said to treat diseases, whereas patients (or people) suffer illnesses. Disease and illness do not necessarily stand in a one-to-one relationship: 70–90 % of all self-recognised episodes of sickness are managed exclusively outside the perimeter of the formal health care system and approximately 50 % of visits to doctors are for complaints without an ascertainable biological basis (27).

Field (op cit) argued that the training of doctors in Western Europe is firmly based on a disease theory of illness. That is, it is based on the assumption that a sound knowledge of the biomedical, chemical and physical processes of health and disease together with the ability to identify correctly the various biological, chemical and physical signs and symptoms of a disease provide a sound base for the practice of medicine. In order to draw attention to, and to make more sense of, the problems of communication between health professionals and the public, sociologists often emphasise the distance between lay and medical beliefs. However, Fitzpatrick (28) argued that those who have stressed this clash of perspectives fail to recognise the major differences that exist between medicine enshrined in textbooks and actual clinical practice. This point will be considered later in the light of Schön's (14) work on "knowing-in-action".

Lock (cited by Fitzpatrick (28)) examined the approaches of medicine to the menopause in the UK. The subject as treated in textbooks is formal, complex and replete with unresolved technical controversies. In reality, Lock found that the views of practising gynaecologists were much simpler and were based on fewer scientific principles. In addition, a range of approaches were taken from the extreme biomedical to the extreme psycho-social. Lock concluded that doctors' views were best understood as folk models to contrast them with formal textual models. Fitzpatrick also cited a study by Gaines that showed that doctors retain many lay assumptions and ideas about illness acquired before training and that these assumptions play an important role in clinical practice alongside formal scientific principles.

General practice may be more directly influenced by lay or folk concepts and can be thought of as a system of thought midway between hospital medicine and lay ideas (29). Marshall Marinker (30) had this to say:

This sort of medicine (whole person medicine) requires from the doctor not only a knowledge of the language and grammar of disease but also of human mythology, a mythology which reaches deep into the origins of the species, the race, and the society. It requires from the doctor an ability to handle the ambiguities and contradictions both of his patient's experience and his own responses.

Helman (29) argued that general practice depends to a large extent on the doctor moving some distance towards the categories that are important to his patient. This is clear, he stated, in the cases of the fevers and colds presented to the general practitioner. Cough mixtures are frequently prescribed even where scientific evidence suggests that they are of negligible value. Yet they do make sense in terms of a folk model that sees cough mixtures as washing out the germs of fevers. Similarly antibiotics are given inappropriately for viral conditions because the doctor is responding to the patient's presentation of "germs" which are not differentiated in the folk model.

Levels and kinds of knowledge

One dimension of knowledge can be expressed as a continuum, from certain and widely agreed knowledge at one end, and at the other end uncertain knowledge that is not generally accepted within countries nor across boundaries, and this includes a lot of mythology and folklore that rigorous scientists might reject as false. Some of this knowledge is stable over time; other knowledge at the growing point is highly volatile, and variable in its diffusion. Steps in the continuum can be described in Table 1 below.

Table 1. Levels of certainty and volatility of biomedical knowledge

Most certain and internationally acceptable:

▲ • Proven and generally accepted knowledge of long standing
| • Knowledge acquired by randomized controlled trials, or widely accepted statistical knowledge
| • Knowledge in rapidly changing fields
| • Rules of thumb – clinical experience and judgement
| • Knowledge of diseases of limited prevalence
| • Unsupported "everyday" knowledge; traditional folklore
| • Medical mythology – diseases that do not exist; totally unsupported
▼   claims to knowledge

Least certain and internationally acceptable knowledge

Knowledge at the head of the list would be predominantly written. Much heuristic knowledge would be locked in the brain of the expert, and the folklore and mythology would be linked to cultural norms and history.

The general practitioner's knowledge must, to some extent, encompass all the categories of knowledge listed above. Much of the knowledge that is required for everyday clinical practice rests within the more uncertain, transient and locally relevant categories in the lower half of the list. Some of this knowledge is a part of, and influenced by, the health beliefs of the population in which the GP practises. However, the core biomedical knowledge required in an international system should be part of the consensus of knowledge within the scientific community. This knowledge will be important for the GP when dealing with the difficult case that might be referred to a specialist. So for life-threatening cases, an international knowledge base might be acceptable, but in order to apply this knowledge in the patient's own cultural setting of illness (as distinct from disease) local knowledge of prevalence and health beliefs would have to be included. This issue brings into focus the essential dilemma of general practice, in attempting to apply rational scientific knowledge and principles in the apparently irrational world of local culture. Computerization of a large knowledge base concentrates the mind on issues of the provenance, reliability and consistency of knowledge. Acceptability of the system will depend on its scientific validity as well as its local acceptability. The computer can easily contain markers as to its provenance and validity, so that general practitioners could have a clearer perception of the level of certainty – whether they were treading on firm ground or quicksand.

For a fully effective knowledge-based system for primary health care, the fringes of uncertain knowledge and cultural determinants of beliefs and behaviour cannot be ignored. However, compromise will be needed in the initial stages of building and validating a decision support system, and a start will have to be made on certain and agreed knowledge. If general practitioners can be helped to solve their increasingly difficult technical problems, as a first step, then attention can later be given to the grey areas of uncertainty and cultural variation. Knowledge-based systems do not need to be as static as a textbook: they can be updated as often as is feasible and affordable.

"Knowing-in-action"

Attempts to apply "artificial intelligence" to professional work have shown how difficult it is to explicate the knowledge of an expert. If asked to explain, the expert will produce a reason for a particular action which rationalizes it, but does not really represent the way the conclusion was reached. "The expert does not think" (31), he or she just knows from experience. This conclusion was also reached by Donald Schön by observing professionals in action, and has been described in "The reflective practitioner" (32) and "Educating the reflective practitioner" (14). Only a fragment of his work can be described here, and the original sources should be consulted.

The knowledge that we use in our work is apparent in our behaviour. The knowing is *in the action*, and is expressed in skilful performance. When trying to reflect upon this knowledge and describe it, we have to give it static structural form as "facts", "procedures", "rules", "values" or "strategies", whereas "knowing-in-action" is spontaneous and responds to a wide variety of stimuli that cannot all be codified. When trying to codify "knowing-in-action" into formal knowledge it loses its spontaneity. Some essential features are listed in Table 2 below:

Table 2   "Knowing-in-action" (from Schön (14))

Knowing is expressed *in the action*
It is spontaneous and dynamic
There is continuous detection and correction of error
Usually the practitioner cannot describe it, except in static terms
May be unrelated to taught professional knowledge
New "knowing-in-action" can be generated from "reflection-in-action"

Much of our daily work is along familiar lines, and we do it "without thinking". The results of earlier thinking have become a habit, so that we can keep going with minimum effort, described by Michael Young (33) as "Habit – the flywheel of society". But every now and again we get a surprise when circumstances do not conform to the pattern that we expected. Do we brush this aside, or do we reflect upon this discrepancy, with the consequent need to revise our "knowing-in-action"? This "stopping to think" is the key to learning, and the continuing gain in knowledge and skills. But it takes time and effort.

Schön (14) described the steps in the process of "reflection-in-action" as in Table 3 below.

Table 3   "Reflection-in action"

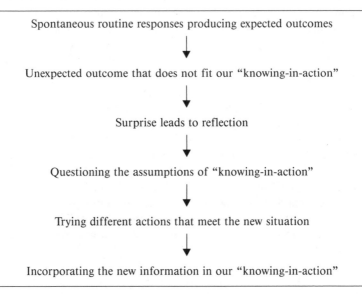

Spontaneous routine responses producing expected outcomes

↓

Unexpected outcome that does not fit our "knowing-in-action"

↓

Surprise leads to reflection

↓

Questioning the assumptions of "knowing-in-action"

↓

Trying different actions that meet the new situation

↓

Incorporating the new information in our "knowing-in-action"

Some professional work is changing so constantly, that nothing comes as a surprise, in which case we have to be on the lookout for "variations". For example, it has been known for over 20 years that the rate of referral of patients to hospital by individual general practitioners has varied by a factor of 5 or more, but only recently have there been serious efforts to find an explanation for these variances. Yet, the implications for patients and for hospital costs are serious. But do we make the time and effort to undertake the reflection, either on the spot, or later when we are in a reflective mood? Timpka and Arborelius (34) have focused the development of a decision support system on the dilemmas experienced in practice, and this seems a fruitful approach which reflects Schön's thinking. These authors' approach to episodes of uncertainty is being integrated into the current Oxford System of Medicine (OSM)/European Community research project on decision support for general practitioners (see section 3).

Individual variations in thinking and reasoning

With a complex decision support architecture as in OSM, many decision paths at many levels are possible. Checking decision paths against outcomes may produce a favoured pathway, but this might not suit all users. People think and reason differently, use different levels of abstraction when relating events to their own model of the world (35), and use different metaphors. Helping people to make decisions in their own way implies a flexibility of operation that is not a characteristic of conventional computer systems. For this flexibility to become a reality, developers and field testers of such a system will have to encompass a wide range of ways of thinking and reasoning. In the case of general practice, consideration would have to be given to the more intuitive and "lateral" approach, rather than the more rigorous reductionist and convergent style associated with scientific medicine.

However, as mentioned earlier, there is a wide gap between theory and practice of medicine, and between the way that experts explain their reasoning and what happens intuitively. The message for builders of KBS is, at least, to keep options open until we have a deeper understanding of the various ways that clinicians work. Provided that there is the built-in audit facility linked to outcome, it should be possible to observe the machine's performance and correct errors continuously. In this way the system could operate in a learning mode, and help the user to do the same.

Gender-linked knowledge

Women's health problems have been the subject of a large number of publications in the past ten years, many of them aimed at women sufferers. At the same time there has been pressure for partnerships of general practitioners in UK to include a woman doctor in the partnership. On the basis of analysis of a large number of video-recorded consultations, the suggestion has been made that women practise medicine differently and that this is more appropriate for their women patients (Sabbagh, K. personal communication). If, in addition to a gender-related knowledge base, there is evidence of gender differences in the application of this knowledge, then a close look must be taken at gender differences in the way knowledge-based systems, and indeed computers are used. If these differences are confirmed, then women (doctors and patients) must be involved in the development of KBS. This approach to "participatory design" (36) does not just relate to gender differences, but to the fundamental principle of involving patients and users in the design of systems at all stages. This is a logical approach to participatory and interdisciplinary learning.

3. What is the current state of development of knowledge-based systems (KBS) for general practice?

A knowledge-based system for general practitioners will need to be integrated with all that conventional systems do now. GPs will only be able to cope with one multi-purpose system, not a different system for each task or domain. It can be assumed, on the basis of current developments (11), that a comprehensive and integrated information and decision support system for general practice will have the following features:

- Very large knowledge base containing around 10 million
- "Facts"[3], coupled to a very large electronic library of textbook and journal information, instantly accessible and up to date (some of it optically stored)
- Patient record system, preferably with intelligent data entry and retrieval (37)
- Logically-programmed decision support function (so-called "expert system")
- Prescribing module, linked with drug and patient information
- Library of approved guidelines, related to patients' preferences, local advice and availability of services
- Audit facility, both "concurrent"[4] and retrospective, linked over time to patient outcomes.

---

3 "Facts" in this context refer to information in a form that a logic program can process, for example "symptoms *of* rheumatoid arthritis *include* joint pain".

4 "Concurrent" audit refers to at process of checking decison options against approved current practice and guidelines, *before* the decision is taken (38). In this way it differs from the usual retrospective audit, which has to be fed back through an educational process and must result in changed behaviour if it is to be effective. Concurrent audit can be achieved with conventional computer programs that include guidelines, but they are likely to be more effective and easier to follow in a knowledge-based decision support system.

The developments outlined above are likely to be feasible within a timescale of three to five years, provided the investment is forthcoming. The main cost would be in developing the very large knowledge base. However, much progress has been made in the past six years and this is outlined below.

The Oxford System of Medicine (OSM) (12) has been under development at the Advanced Computation Laboratory, Imperial Cancer Research Fund in London, with some input from the Oxford University Press. The current state of the "demonstrator" is outlined below:

- A knowledge base of around 20,000 "facts" plus the Oxford Textbook of Medicine (2e) on CD ROM (39), integrated into OSM
- Patient record system in OSM under development (PEN and PAD (37), uses advanced "intelligent" data retrieval)
- Generic decision support software is functional (40)
- Work is in hand on the inclusion of information from the British National Formulary and the Monthly Index of Medical Specialities, and the development of an electronic practice formulary
- Guidelines program under development, with colleagues in Oxford and the Netherlands
- Audit module not yet developed.

The plan is for practices to have a distributed "stand-alone" system that would use a conventional 386 microcomputer, with a graphical interface and mouse, and a compact disk reader. Networking would not be essential, though it could make communication with hospitals easier, for referral appointments, and two-way transfer of information.

Following a successful research programme funded by the European Commission in 1990 (AIM)[5], work has started on a major second phase of research and development as part of the AIM (1991–1994) programme.

Compiling a very large knowledge base of 10 million "facts" is certain to give rise to problems of knowledge representation and classification. In order to produce a single, generalist knowledge base using knowledge from many specialties, problems of compatibility and nomenclature will have to be faced. In addition, there are few hard data about the information needs of general practitioners. All these topics are the subject of active research.

---

5 Advanced Informatics in Medicine.

Though progress to date has been promising, and sound principles have been developed, the Oxford System of Medicine (OSM) still has to be evaluated in practice and shown to be acceptable in everyday use. Indeed, proof is still needed that decision support in medicine does lead to improved outcomes for patients and to professional learning. At least, the OSM should be able to provide the answers (see section 4 (v)).

The Oxford System of Medicine, though primarily aimed at general practitioners, could well be helpful to junior doctors in hospital training posts, and also to specialists having the care of patients with problems outside their specialist domain.

4. Can the effectiveness of the process of referral of patients to hospital be improved by knowledge-based systems?

As argued above, general practitioners need to take on as wide a generalist role as possible, and in the UK they are able to look after 90 % of episodes of illness. Yet about 10 % of consultations end in referral to a hospital specialist (41). These include the more seriously ill patients and the effectiveness of referral is a key issue in providing cost-effective health care. Yet the variances in referral rates are not fully explained (42). Is it possible that referral could become more effective if general practitioners had access to more appropriate knowledge (about the patient, about biomedicine and about policies and availability of services), and also had help in ordering the options and coming to a better decision?

The general practitioner's bridging role

One of the purposes of referral is to give the patient the benefit of the specialist's superior knowledge in a particular domain. The level of the general practitioner's knowledge in that domain is an important factor in the referral decision (43). If referral is needed, then the more knowledgeable GP will have a better grasp of which specialist is appropriate and what the specialist can offer. In addition, the referral letter could contain information that is more relevant to the specialist's task. The GP will have to explore the extent of the patient's knowledge and beliefs, and make this information available to the specialist, where relevant. Another advantage of narrowing the knowledge gap between GP and specialist relates to levels of assumed or "tacit" knowledge that is shared. The same applies to the knowledge gap between GP and patient. The general practitioner has the Herculean task of spanning an ever widening knowledge gap, and interpreting patient's knowledge and concerns to the specialist, and vice versa. The GP can be helped, at the interface with the patient, by other members of the primary health care team, some of whom may have closer rapport with the patient.

How might knowledge-based decision support systems improve the quality of the referral process?

(i)   Making relevant and up-to-date knowledge available to the GP on screen, during the consultation

First and foremost, the general practitioner could obtain knowledge, relevant to the context, available instantly as needed and in a concise form. This knowledge would be about patients, about biomedicine and about locally agreed procedures and availability of services. The less volatile and more certain knowledge could be available on a stack of compact discs, using existing technology. More volatile knowledge could be updated on disk or on-line. Many such systems exist using "slab text" and "hypertext" on a conventional computer. In the UK there is "Pandora" (Longmore, M. personal communication) and in Finland the Physician's Desk Reference and Database (PDRD), (Kunnamo, I. personal communication). The Oxford System of Medicine uses these methods and integrates them with the built-in logically-structured knowledge base. The user can browse around the system, like in a library, but can get much quicker access to data with "intelligent" search programs which search for meanings not just words and their associations.

(ii)   Helping to fill in relevant gaps in the data, e.g. history, signs and tests

Knowledge-based information support has the potential advantage that data relevant to the immediate problem can be automatically selected and incorporated in the decision support process. This should make it much easier and quicker to use in practice. In addition, the system can highlight missing patient data that is relevant to the current problem. By doing this while the patient is present, the missing data can often be found, automatically recorded in the patient record and incorporated in the logical inferences. For example, in a case of joint pain[6], the GP is prompted to enquire about alopecia. If present, this provides supporting evidence for a diagnosis of systemic lupus erythematosus. In this way a difficult case can have a more thorough and logical "work-up" before a decision on referral or treatment is taken.

Diagnostic possibilities can be listed in a tree structure. Where there is support for a diagnosis, this is starred. Several options are displayed and weighted according to the number of supporting factors. Statistical tests of probabilities are not applied at this stage of development as numerical data relevant to general practice are largely non-existent. Tests that might refine the diagnosis can also be listed, and the evidence weighed up. Missing data are queried and treatment possibilities are listed.

The GP using the system has to make the final choice about diagnosis, investigation, treatment and/or referral. The system can only support the doctor's decisions, not make them. The reasoning process must be transparent, so that at any point the doctor can ask why a particular statement appeared on the screen.

(iii) Prescribing support, integrated with decision support

Conventional programs exist for helping the GP prescribe safely and effectively. Their power and selectivity could be greatly enhanced in the setting of a system such as OSM, with the result that the doctor is more likely to use the checking program, rather than ignore or disable it. If the incidence of iatrogenic disease could be reduced, then this would affect referrals beneficially. The litigation element might also be reduced.

(iv) Helping the GP to conform to accepted guidelines

Though this is a controversial area, the use of guidelines for investigation, treatment and referral in medicine as a whole is gaining support (44). Guidelines encapsulate a very large amount of written knowledge and expertise, or "knowing-in-action", in a small compass. To do this, without endless qualifications, means that there must be compromise, with the result that circumstances arise in which the guidelines cannot be applied. Sometimes this may happen because the guidelines are faulty and not based on all the available evidence. Eddy (45) sounded a timely warning against guidelines produced by a group of people who describe existing practice as the ideal, rather

---

6 The OSM demonstrator contained seven test cases taken from examination questions of the Royal College of Physicians of London.

than examine all the evidence. He dismisses the former as tautological. Eddy's ideal is the guideline based on outcomes for patients, coupled with an option to allow for patient preferences, but admits that these hardly exist. Exceptions are, perhaps, in the field of perinatal illness (46) and the guidelines produced by the Royal College of Radiologists. The Dutch College of General Practitioners has produced a number of guidelines for general practitioners that are gaining acceptance. The OSM group have studied some of these guidelines and, in cooperation with specialist colleagues in Oxford, are developing a decision support program for treatment and referral of lipid disorders[7], asthma, colorectal cancers and diabetes. The aim is not just to help the individual practitioner's decision making, but also to make shared care more effective.

As mentioned earlier, it must be possible to integrate such modules into a comprehensive decision support system, not just to have a series of stand-alone modules. When guidelines fail or cannot be applied, the user is left in a quandary. However, when such guidelines are part of a comprehensive system, it can always be used to provide further decision support, taking into account the factors that have caused the formal guideline to fail.

(v) Providing automatic audit, both concurrently and retrospectively

As mentioned earlier, a knowledge-based decision support system can produce an instant "audit" of conformity of decision options to guidelines or to the larger body of medical knowledge. Over time, an "audit trail" of its use can be logged and related to the patient's subsequent progress. In this way, by linking the decisions to outcomes for patients, it should be possible to measure the quality and effectiveness of the decision process itself, as well as the guidelines. This opens up new possibilities for improving the quality of care of patients, and also for building up a body of medical knowledge that is based directly on patient outcomes in general practice. This would allow doctors to answer two critical questions that are rarely addressed in general practice, namely:

Is the intervention likely to do good, taking into account all the available evidence?
Has the intervention actually benefited the patient, without unacceptable side-effects?

---

7 Widespread population screening for lipid disorders sharpens the need for referral to be more selective, if lipid clinics are not to be overwhelmed.

One of the failings of the present arrangements for knowledge transfer is that much of the new knowledge is generated in specialist fields using referred patients. This knowledge must be validated in the very different context of general practice before it can be relied upon. Pooled, anonymous data from decision support systems could achieve a new integration of specialist medicine and general practice, which could be the basis for a very different pattern of referral practices from those that are in use today.

(vi) Reducing uncertainty, with a consequent increase in GPs' confidence and self-esteem

As described earlier, GPs have to work under conditions of great uncertainty, in which it is tempting just to get by on what can be remembered, rather than engage in a process of interaction with a very large knowledge base. From this interaction, learning is bound to flow, because the knowledge is relevant to the immediate problem (47). Professions have traditionally relied on exclusive knowledge as a source of power (48). Today, the information revolution has made medical knowledge more accessible to patients, but at the same time, the very quantity of available knowledge has overwhelmed many GPs. New generations of computer systems could go a long way towards restoring the role of general practitioners as knowledge brokers, and consequently raising their confidence to support a more effective level of performance.

(vii) Longer term effects of decision support on the referral process.

A major challenge such as the impact of knowledge-based computer systems on general practice can be seen both as a threat and as an opportunity. Will general practitioners accept the new systems, or retreat into a backwater of providing emotional support, cut off from the mainstream of knowledge? A recent pilot study of 177 GPs, mostly members of educational networks, in nine European countries (15) was reassuring, in that the great majority saw the value of such systems and welcomed them. In particular, they favoured easy access to medical and drug information, screening, prescribing and information about specialist clinics. Referral decision support was less popular, though the majority were in favour.

Keeping referral to a minimum might be seen as desirable for the convenience of patients and for minimizing costs, but the optimum referral level may be higher than current average levels. Decision support could provide a clearer formulation of policies for referral and shared care. If the implementation of these policies cannot be afforded, then a rational rethinking of the boundaries between primary and secondary care, based on better information, would be essential. Any change in the boundary between GP and specialist would raise the issue of altered knowledge needs which would have to be met by educational means.

Referral has been considered at length, as the whole topic is surrounded in mystery, and yet it is crucial that referral and shared care should work optimally, both for the benefit of the patient and for ensuring that health services, with their limited funding, can use resources where they produce most benefit in human and medical terms.

5. What impact might KBS have on patients' knowledge and on communication in the consultation?

Specific information is mostly transmitted in the consultation by the spoken word, but also non-verbally by eye contact, body language and a variety of other visual and non-visual cues (49). As mentioned earlier, there are advantages in viewing the patients as experts, who can contribute not only the medical history, but also their beliefs and aspirations and their view of the world in which they live and to which they have to adapt. In addition, they have specific knowledge and experience about their health and about health in general, even if this is dismissed by professionals as folklore. We can all quote examples where doctors' empathy and effectiveness are greatly increased when they have suffered from a particular disease.

Patients need information about their illness and its management, from whatever source they find best and easiest to access and understand, supported by explanation of causes and prevention where possible. In addition they need explanation and dialogue about what their illness might entail for their own and their family's feelings and future well-being. This requires a level of understanding and empathy which could be a part of the general practitioner's role. Research has shown that general practitioners are good at explanation when asked by the patient, but rarely offer the deeper level of explanation based on empathic understanding (9). Whether knowledge-based systems would help or hinder this deeper level of communication is another open question. Transfer of information is clearly linked to patient satisfaction and compliance (6), and so should benefit both doctor and patient. But as well as pragmatic reasons for giving information, there is the conviction that giving information reduces the patient's uncertainty. However, in doing so the doctor reduces his own power (50). These authors also showed that doctors underestimate patients' level of knowledge, and as a consequence communicate less information. Patients' expectations are rising as consumers gain in knowledge and confidence, though there is the countervailing trend of cost containment which could lead to an acceptance of poor standards of care. Inequity may thereby increase, as there is clear evidence that those in social classes 4 and 5 may fare less well in their utilization of information and in their uptake of health care. This puts an onus on doctors to take the initiative in providing clear information for all their patients – about health, illness and treatment, about keeping well, about the practice and about rights to health care. Whether the introduction of a knowledge-based system to the consultation will increase inequity is an open question which must be addressed. The salutary lesson is that doctors must function as leaders in giving more rather than less information, and must be prepared to sacrifice the power based on the secrecy of professional knowledge, in exchange for the benefits to all of a more open and equal relationship.

When patients have a specific disability such as diabetes or cystic fibrosis, and are in touch with a self-help group, they may well know more about the problems of coping with the illness than the general practitioner or even the specialist. There are now over 1000 self-help groups related to health in the UK (51). Some are developing extensive databases for patients and professionals to use, so cooperation and compatibility of knowledge as well as technology need to be addressed, if the patient is not to be presented with two conflicting sources of knowledge.

As a first step, the importance of the patient's knowledge, including "knowing-in-action" can be recognized. The next step will be to explore the nature and extent of this "patient-specific" knowledge, and turn it to good use. To do this requires close cooperation with self-help groups related to health. There is no reason why this knowledge should not be available to patient and professional alike in a knowledge-based system. The main barrier to its implementation is likely to be the reluctance of doctors to have patients who are better informed than themselves (52). But already the tide of public knowledge has bypassed any professional dams: will the doctor's role as a source of knowledge and explanation also be bypassed? Patients remember little of what they are told in the consultation (6), so knowledge based computer systems might fill the gap by producing written material suited to the patient's needs and circumstances.

Knowledge-based decision support systems, with their initial need to concentrate on the more certain areas of biomedical knowledge, may well fail to meet these requirements. Whether they will distract the doctor from areas of patient knowledge, or by removing some of the anxieties arising from lack of technical knowledge, they may help the doctor to concentrate on patients' problems of adapting to illness, remain open questions. Much of the knowledge now available to patients is difficult for the lay person to understand and evaluate, and much is communicated one-way, rather than as part of a dialogue. A possible role for the doctor could be to guide the patient through this Aladdin's cave, but this can only succeed if the doctor really understands the patient's knowledge needs. Maybe a specialist librarian could do it, or a member of a self-help group. The threat to professional survival will remain, unless doctors and their patients can both access the relevant knowledge and help each other to apply it in the unique circumstances of the consultation.

6. What impact might KBS have on professional learning and education, particularly as regards communication of knowledge?

Much of what has gone before is relevant to learning, but in this section the focus will be more on the way general practitioners gain and maintain knowledge. At a basic pragmatic level, medical students and practitioners will have to have the necessary skills to operate (not program) computer systems. A system like OSM will require a considerable change in working method in the consultation, and for this intensive training and continuing support will be needed. The methods of concurrent audit are revolutionary, and will need attitudinal change. They will, however, operate almost automatically, so that time spent on laborious retrospective audit and re-education could be replaced by learning in other areas, such as skills, or spent on learning by "reflection-in-action".

At present, general practitioners in the UK go on refresher courses on a variety of self-selected topics. The topics are likely to be those in which the GP is interested and knows well, rather than focusing on areas of poor performance. Many refresher courses aim to impart knowledge about new treatments, but this knowledge would be much more appropriately contributed at the moment it was needed in the consultation, as OSM would achieve. Though this knowledge need not be a burden on the doctor's memory, in practice the "hot" learning situation might provide more effective learning, as Sackett and colleagues (47) have emphasized.

Though it is hard to predict the effects on learning of powerful tools like knowledge-based decision support, they will certainly not be trivial. For example, if factual knowledge that can be expressed in text is easily available in the system, then there can be more emphasis on the development of "knowing-in-action" and "reflection-in-action" as described earlier. In addition, there will be more time for learning skills, both manual therapeutic skills and communication skills. Computer-aided instruction and computer-assisted learning have found little favour in medical teaching in the UK, and in the educational world as a whole (53). However, knowledge-based systems are designed as "aids to doing" one's everyday work, not specifically directed at learning. There is evidence that the use of simple decision-support systems, for example for the diagnosis of the cause of abdominal pain (54), do improve diagnostic performance even when the user has ceased to use the decision aid, but evidence of this decay of learning is conflicting.

Medical teachers and educationists who look ahead, in this case over the horizon, will find it hard to predict what the professional's job will be like ten or twenty years hence: equally unpredictable will be the learning methods and tools that the new information technology will make available. More immediately, teachers will need to ensure that students and practitioners are equipped with the skills to cope with major developments in information technology. One such strategic approach has been adopted by the University of Calgary in their curriculum on medical informatics for under-graduate medical students (Jennett, P. personal communication), which allows space for learning about knowledge-based systems when they arrive.

In spite of the pioneer work of people like Elstein and colleagues (55) and Gale and Marsden (56), our understanding of medical problem solving and diagnosis is not very profound. As a consequence, it is difficult to design and build a decision support system that has any relationship to these activities in real life. This leaves us with the option to build an empirical tool that will aim to improve outcomes for patients. The way the decision support system is used can leave an "audit trail" which can be linked to outcomes for patients. In time this would allow us to learn what interventions and what decision processes are likely to have the better outcomes, even if we do not understand why this was so. Decision support systems linked to "intelligent" medical records present us with the opportunity for much more systematic learning by experience. By so doing, practitioners will have a more objective measure of the value of the services provided to balance against the cost. Value for money in health care is a sensible objective, but when measures of quality are lacking, cost and *quantity* of care tend to be the yardsticks.

With knowledge becoming more widespread and accessible to the public through electronic means, the role of the doctor is changing from being the fount of traditional knowledge, towards being a catalyst who brings about a reaction between knowledge and the patient (with the catalyst's advantage of not being destroyed in the process). An educational system that regards itself as a fount of knowledge will be unlikely to succeed, so we may need to look towards more interactive learning, in which the patient is also a teacher and the computer a mirror to guide our steps and log our performance.

An approach to adapting to fundamental change that is becoming popular in industry and the public services is to develop a "learning organization" (57), and for all those involved in the organization to "operate in a learning mode" as part of their everyday behaviour (58). This has a parallel with individual self-directed learning, but on the level of the care group including the patient (59). By this means the learning process becomes an essential part of daily behaviour, supported by the organization, so that it is seen as part of corporate identity. To ensure that this is happening, there is a need to evaluate both individual and organizational learning – termed "double-loop learning". This is a particular province of the educationist – to evaluate what learning is happening, and keep it going. This is a very different process from identifying and filling gaps in knowledge, and represents another example of the "catalyst" model.

7. What future prospects are likely, and what is the balance of costs and benefits of implementing advanced information technology?

It is too late to ask the question "Will the information technology revolution affect medicine and medical education?". The lesson of history is that technological changes cannot be resisted, so we need to rephrase the questions to "when and how will it happen?", "what are the benefits and costs?", and "how can we maximize the benefits at minimum cost in material, social and psychological terms?" (17, 60, 61).

Traditionally, the costs and benefits are weighed up purely in economic terms relating to the efficiency, effectiveness and utility of the process or sub-process concerned, with scant regard to human systems, both in relation to the operators of the new system (health professionals) and the presumed beneficiary (the patient). At the design stage, technological issues tend to outweigh the needs of the users and the patients' needs and preferences are ignored. Lip service may be paid to their needs, but unless users and patients are involved in the design process, their underlying needs and beliefs will be forgotten until it is too late. In addition, their involvement at the design stage can be creative. This reluctance to involve "consumers" in the active development and management of services aimed to benefit them is a shortcoming of nearly all health care and education systems.

A possible future scenario of a revitalized health care system, incorporating knowledge-based decision support, could perhaps be along these lines.

The patient with a symptom that caused anxiety would first consult the "home doctor" program incorporated in their television set. This would reveal a number of options and anxieties that the system could not resolve, so the patient would contact their general practitioner by telephone or preferably videophone, with shared information on the patient's and the GP's screens. If, with the benefit of the biographical record, an extensive knowledge base, enquiries of the patient and even some self examination, the problem could not be resolved, then a visit to the general practitioner might be needed.

The consultation would follow the traditional model of enquiry set out by Pendleton et al. (5) by defining the history, nature and cause of the problem; exploring the patient's ideas, concerns and expectations; exploring the effects of problems, continuing problems and risk factors; appropriate action chosen and a shared understanding and involvement of the patient achieved; and a helpful relationship established and maintained.

This could all be supported by the knowledge-based system providing prompts and summaries of weighted options, with the doctor and patient working through the problem together, with contributions from both. Intervention, such as referral or a prescription could be negotiated against the background of consensus medical knowledge or agreed guidelines, where available.

The doctor's role in helping the patient who felt unwell, but did not show evidence of physical disease, could be enhanced by the knowledge that the physical problem had been thoroughly explored together.

The potential benefit of the thoroughness that a knowledge-based system can provide must be balanced by the time it takes to work through the system, and the potential for distraction away from the social and psychological issues that might not be incorporated in the knowledge base. The general practitioner might be tempted to become a machine-minder who ignored issues outside the machine. Conversely GPs might enhance their potential to help with non-physical illness, by nature of the confidence that their technical mastery engenders. In other words they would gain an enhanced healing power.

The scenario described could go astray in a number of ways, and competition for attention between the new "machine operator" role, and the traditional empathic role might be inevitable, if only because of time pressure. More seriously would be the tendency of computer support to direct the GP to the technical end of the behavioural spectrum, as against being patient-oriented when appropriate (3).

The educational needs of the new-style GP would be very different, both because of the very different style of working, but also because the development of knowledge-based technology will alter the whole structure of the medical knowledge base, will "dynamise" its use by virtue of concurrent audit, and will alter the face of medicine and its impact on patients and society. Doctors, educationists, computer scientists and patients will have to cooperate at the design, implementation and evaluation stages to ensure that the technology retains a human purpose and a human face.

References

1. What sort of doctor? Assessing quality of care in general practice. Report from General Practice. London: Royal College of General Practitioners, 1985.
2. Cartwright A, Anderson R. General Practice revisited. A second study of patients and their doctors. London: Tavistock Publications, 1981.
3. Byrne P, Long B. Doctors talking to patients. A study of the verbal behaviour of general practitioners consulting in their surgeries. London: HMSO, 1976. Republished by Royal College of General Practitioners, 1989.
4. Balint M. The doctor, his patient and the illness. Revised second edition. London: Pitman Medical, 1964.
5. Pendleton D, Schofield T, Tate P, Havelock P. The consultation. An approach to learning and teaching. Oxford: Oxford University Press, 1984.

6. Ley P. Communicating with patients. Improving communication, satisfaction and compliance. London: Croom Helm, 1989.
7. King J. Health beliefs in the consultation. In: Pendleton D, Hasler J, eds. Doctor-patient communication. London: Academic Press, 1983.
8. Harris TA. I'm OK – you're OK. London: Pan books, 1967 (reprint edition 1973).
9. Tuckett D et al. Meeting between experts. An approach to sharing ideas in medical consultations. London: Tavistock, 1985.
10. Pritchard PMM. The information avalanche. Can the general practitioner survive? Practitioner 1985; 229: 877-81.
11. Fox J et al. Logic engineering for knowledge engineering: design and implementation of the Oxford System of Medicine. Artificial Intelligence in Medicine 1990, 2: 323-39.
12. Gordon C et al. The design of the Oxford System of Medicine: an overview. In O'Moore RO et al., eds. Lecture notes in medical informatics, Vol 40, Berlin: Springer-Verlag, 1991.
13. Pritchard, PMM. The role of computers in referral. In Hopkins A, Wallace P, eds. Referral to medical outpatients. London: Royal College of Physicians, 1992.
14. Schön DA. Educating the reflective practitioner. Towards a new design for teaching and learning in the professions. San Francisco: Jossey-Bass, 1990.
15. Ginzler M, Pritchard PMM. Can medical knowledge-based systems cross frontiers? The Oxford System of Medicine in the context of trans-national markets. Report to the European Commission. AIM project 1024. London: Advanced Computation Laboratory, Imperial Cancer Research Fund, 1990.
16. Haynes RB et al. A critical appraisal of the efficacy of continuing medical education. JAMA 1984; 251:61-4.
17. Cooley M. The new technology and the new training. Reflections on the past and prospects for the future. In Göranzon B, Florin M, eds. Artificial intelligence, culture and language: on education and work. London: Springer-Verlag 1990.
18. Abel-Smith B. Cost containment in health care. A study of 12 European countries. Occasional papers on social administration No 73. London: Bedford Square Press, 1984.
19. WHO/UNICEF The Alma Ata Declaration. Geneva: WHO, 1978.
20. Weiss P. Health and biomedical information in Europe. Copenhagen: WHO Regional Office for Europe, 1986.
21. Sandor L et al. A survey of the distribution of the world oncological publications from 1969-1974. Zeitschrift für Krebsforschung 1976; 86: 209-18.
22. Jacobs W. Deutschlands Ärztefortbildung: Überblick, Kritik und Anregungen. Der Deutsche Arzt; 27: 30-50.
23. Stross JK, Harlan WR. The dissemination of new medical information. JAMA 1979; 241: 2622-4.
24. Gillie A. Reflections on the Gillie report. J R Coll Gen Pract 1964; 7: 1-8.
25. Barley S. The literature of general practice. In Westcott R, Jones RVH, eds. Information handling in general practice. London: Croom Helm, 1988.
26. Field D. The social definition of illness. In Tuckett D, ed. An introduction to medical sociology. London: Tavistock, 1976.
27. Kleinman A et al. Culture, illness and care: clinical lessons from anthropologic and cross-cultural research. J Intern Med 1978; 88: 251-8.
28. Fitzpatrick R. The experience of illness. London: Tavistock, 1984.
29. Helman C. Culture, health and illness, 2nd edition. Bristol: Wright, 1990.
30. Marinker M. The chameleon, the judas goat and the cuckoo. J R Coll Gen Pract 1978; 28:199-206.
31. Dreyfus HL. Is Socrates to blame for cognitivism? In: Göranzon B, Florin M, eds. Artificial intelligence, culture and language. On education and work. London: Springer-Verlag, 1990
32. Schön DA. The reflective practitioner. New York: Basic Books, 1983.

33. Young M. The metronomic society. Natural rhythms and human timetables. London: Thames and Hudson, 1988.
34. Timpka T, Arborelius E. The GP's dilemmas. A study of knowledge need and use during health care consultations. Methods Inf Med 1990; 29: 23-9.
35. Gaines BR, Shaw MLG. A learning model for forecasting the future of information technology. Future Computing Systems 1986; 1: 31-69.
36. Gill K. Cultures, language, mediation. In: Göranzon B, Florin M, eds. Artificial intelligence, Culture and language. On education and work. London: Springer-Verlag, 1990.
37. Nolan W, Rector A, Kaye S. 'Pen & Pad' a doctors workstation with intelligent data entry and summaries. Washington DC: SCAMC 90, 1990.
38. Pritchard P. Can decision making be improved? Postgraduate Education for General Practice 1991, 2: 4-6.
39. Oxford Textbook of Medicine (2nd edition) on compact disk. Oxford: Oxford Electronic Publishing, Oxford University Press, 1989.
40. Clarke DA, Fox J, Glowinski AJ, O'Neil MJ. Symbolic reasoning for decision making. In: Borcherding K, Larichov OL, Messick DM, eds. Contemporary issues in decision making. Amsterdam: Elsevier Science Publications BV, 1989.
41. Fowler G. Primary health care. In: Weatherall D, Ledingham JGG, Warrell DA, eds. Oxford Textbook of Medicine (2nd edition). Oxford: Oxford University Press, 1987.
42. Coulter A, Roland M, Wilkin D. GP referrals to hospital. A guide for Family Health Services Authorities. Manchester: Center for primary care research, Department of General Practice, 1991.
43. Hutchinson A, Hayes V, Newton J. Factors influencing general practitioner referral decisions. Newcastle: Health Care Research Unit, Newcastle upon Tyne, 1990.
44. Woolf SM. Practice Guidelines: A new realitly in medicine. Arch Intern Med 1990; 150: 1811-18.
45. Eddy DM. Designing a Practice Policy. Standards, Guidelines and Options. JAMA 1990; 263: 3077-84.
46. Chalmers I, ed. Oxford Database of Perinatal Trials. Oxford: Oxford Electronic Publishing, Oxford University Press, 1989.
47. Sackett DL et al. Clinical epidemiology: a basic science for clinical medicine. Boston and Toronto: Little Brown and Co, 1985.
48. Hughes E. The Study of Occupations. In: Merton RK, Broom L, Cottrell LS Jr, eds. Sociology Today. New York: Basic Books, 1959.
49. Argyle M. Doctor-patient skills. In: Pendleton D, Hasler J, eds. Doctor-Patient Communication. London: Academic Press, 1983.
50. Waitzkind H, Stoeckle JD. The communication of information about illness. Adv Psychosom Med 1972; 8: 108-215.
51. Gann R. The health information handbook, resources for self-care. Aldershot: Gower, 1986.
52. Westcott R. A review of information for people. In: Westcott R, Jones RVH, eds. Information handling in general practice: challenges for the future. London: Croom Helm, 1988.
53. Beveridge M. Educational implications of intelligent systems. In: Murray LA, Richardson JTE, eds. Intelligent systems in a human context. Oxford: Oxford University Press, 1989.
54. de Dombal FT et al. Human and computer aided diagnosis of abdominal pain: further report with emphasis on performance of clinicians. BMJ 1974; 1: 376-80.
55. Elstein AS, Schulman LS, Sprafka SA. Medical problems solving: an analysis of clinical reasoning. Cambridge, Mass.: Harvard University Press, 1978.
56. Gale J, Marsden P. Medical diagnosis. From student to clinician. Oxford: Oxford University Press, 1983.

57. Argyris C, Schön DA. Organizational learning: a theory of action perspective. Reading, Mass.: Addison-Wesley, 1978.
58. Beckhard R, Pritchard W. Changing the essence: the art of creating and leading fundamental change in organizations. San Francisco: Jossey-Bass, 1992.
59. Pritchard PMM, Pritchard JR. Developing teamwork in primary health care. A practical workbook. Practical guides for general practice No 15. Oxford: Oxford University Press, 1992.
60. Finne H. (How) can technology be redirected? A Scandinavian perspective. In: Rosenbrock HH, ed. Designing human-centered technology, London: Springer-Verlag, 1989.
61. Ennals R. Artificial Intelligence and Human Institutions. Berlin: Springer-Verlag, 1991.

9

Reading and Writing in the Learning of Medicine

RICHARD SMITH

"It is astonishing with how little reading a doctor can practice medicine, but it is not astonishing how badly he may do it."

Sir William Osler, 1849-1919 (1)

Reading and writing are not only two of the most ancient tools of learning but they are also two of the tools first used by children. Surely, we might think in a moment of modernistic excess, such methods cannot be so important in teaching medicine, which depends so much today on modern technology. Now that we have interactive computers, videos, role playing, spreadsheets, algorithms, television, and a dozen other up to the minute methods of learning we shouldn't have much need of those two ancient tools of reading and writing. But almost nobody could be found to sustain such an argument. Reading and writing are indispensable in learning medicine today.

The two great assets of reading are that it offers vast depth and breadth within a tiny human sized space – a page – and that it allows every student a chance to make his or her own journey. Libraries contain the whole world. In time they range from the first beginnings to the farthest future, and in space they stretch from inside the atom to the whole universe and beyond. And in style and philosophy libraries may include everything from the intimacy and poetry of mystical writing to the hardest of data. With such vastness available for free and without need to travel physically the student can make a journey that within seconds will be different from that made by any other student ever. He or she can go as far and as fast as he or she wants – flying across centuries or creeping into ants' burrows. And he or she can go backwards or forwards, checking and confirming, questioning and exploring, following any path that might appeal.

I may begin to sound silly in this paragraph that I have just
written, but I want to try and remind readers of the magic that we
may be taking for granted. We may think of libraries as dull, sleepy
places and librarians as boring people, but a good library is one of
the places on earth where we can come closest to paradise. The South
American writer, Jorge Luis Borges, captures the excitement and
mystery of a great library in his story "The library of Babel." He
compares the library to the universe:

> ... the Library is total... its shelves register ... all that it is given
> to express, in all languages. Everything: the minutely detailed
> history of the future, the archangels' biographies, the faithful
> catalogue of the Library, thousands and thousands of false cata-
> logues, the demonstration of the fallacy of those catalogues, the
> Gnostic bible of Basilides, the commentary on that gospel, the
> commentary on the commentary on that gospel, the true story of
> your death, the translation of every book in all languages, the
> interpolations of every book in all books" (2).

Sir William Osler was more prosaic but no less inspired in what he
had to say about the usefulness of the library for a doctor: "For the
general practitioner, a well used library is one of the few correctives
of the premature senility which is so apt to overtake him" (1).

Writing is, I think, essential for two qualities: it forces you to be
clear about what you think; and the very process of writing allows
discovery. One of the most exciting events in writing a novel is when
characters take on a life of their own and begin to take unexpected
actions. The same may happen in much less ambitious forms of writing: as students write their essays on biochemistry they may discover
quite new connections or patterns that may help to make sense of
what at times seems an impenetrable subject.

A philosophy of education

Before expanding further on how I think reading and writing are crucially important in the learning of medicine I want – in order to develop my case – to say something about my philosophy of education.
I want to begin by quoting something that I wrote when I was 15 and
"suffering" from education in a way that at times seemed terminal.
I wrote the piece for a competition organised by the British newspaper "The Observer." Some of the many thousands of entries were

collected in a book called "The school that I'd like" (3). In 1967 I wrote:

> What's he droning on about? Africa. What the hell's that like?
> Does it look like that line of dustbins through the window? Does it feel like this inkwell? Does it sound like that traffic or this continuous drone? Does it smell like carbolic soap? Does it taste like this bubblegum?
> What is the answer to this dreaming atmosphere of the classroom? There are several, but the simplest and yet overlooked one is to get rid of classrooms. Instead of stuffing children into a classroom, within four boundaries. let them get out and see, feel, smell, hear and taste the subject. Bring it alive.

I was writing about the boredom of British education, and I was not alone. The editor, Edward Blishen, wrote:

> ... one of the discoveries made by all those who read the essays was that a few schools seem able to set their children free, intellectually, while others, having children of the same calibre and capacity, shut them up in the prison of a most dreadful conformity... The picture they [the children] build up of learning as it is now most often in the schools is one in which they, the pupils, are passive, sometimes very reluctant, recipients; the teachers are the providers ... It is this pattern of passively receiving, magisterially providing, that children worry away at... From all the quarters of the educational scene it comes, this expression of children's longing to take upon themselves some of the burden of deciding what should be learnt, how it should be learnt; this desire to get closer to the raw matter of learning, not to be presented with predigested knowledge by teacher...

All I can say is that when I arrived in Edinburgh Medical School in 1970 it was worse. And Edinburgh was not alone. In July 1991 a professor of general practice wrote in the BMJ about medical schools boring their students rigid (4), and the result was a tremendous ahmen (sic). Reading allows a thousand routes of escape from the prison of boring education – if the students have the time and skills to find them.

Another important ingredient of my philosophy of education I learnt not from an educator but from the president of one of the world's largest computer companies – Jean Louis Gassee of Apple. He illustrated learning with figure 1 and described it as a matter of matching challenge with skills. To learn effectively we must move up the line that intersects the axes of challenge and skills. But reality will not be so smooth: instead we will snake up the line. We will sometimes be in circumstances where the challenges will exceed our skills, leading to anxiety, but at other times our skills will exceed the challenge, leading to boredom. Education must contain both challenges and opportunities to enhance skills, and reading and writing can supply both.

Monsieur Gassee also had an interesting response when asked whether computers might bring about a revolution in education. "Educational programmes on computers are nothing more," he said, "than electronic flash cards. Computers will not think for 20 years because intelligence is born out of desire and computers have no desire. You only learn when you lust after learning. Computers have no dark side, and it is the dark side of men and women that is the interesting side. Creativity comes out of the tensions created by greed, evil, jealousy, despair and all the other dark emotions that computers don't possess." Perhaps he got carried away, but he is making strongly the point that education is not just a matter of neatly filling up sunny students with all the skills and knowledge they need. It is a messy business – like life itself – and there must be room for passion. Medical schools are thin on passion, but libraries are full of passion.

Education must then, I believe, contain excitement, and it must encourage and reward insatiable curiosity and a lust for learning. Educators should thus accept students making their own journeys down paths that they, the educators, may not approve. Indeed, they should encourage such journeys, and they may impart this through something that Walter Bagehot, a great 19th century editor described as awe. "A schoolmaster," he wrote, "should have an atmosphere of awe, and walk wonderingly, as if he was amazed at being himself." Awe is a somewhat old-fashioned word, associated primarily with religion, but its definition gives clues to what I believe are some of the keys of education. "Awe," says Webster's dictionary, "is an overwhelming feeling of reverence, admiration, fear, etc. produced by that which is grand, sublime, extremely powerful or the like." But students should not feel awe for the institutions of medicine; rather they should feel awe for the unending pursuit for better methods of increasing health and reducing disease that is at the heart of medicine.

Successful education will also be fun in the sense understood by children. If it is nothing but unremitting dreariness then students – like children – will turn their attention elsewhere. But at the same time an essential characteristic of those who learn successfully is "stickability," which might also be described as persistence and assiduity. Learning does not always come easily; indeed, most of it comes hard. "One learns nothing by reading," said one Oxford don, "but only by rereading."

Another vital component of the learning process must be encouragement to question everything, particularly dogma and received wisdom. "The surest way to corrupt a young man,"said the German philosopher, Friedrich Nietzsche, "is to teach him to esteem more highly those who think alike than those who think differently." Critical questioning is at the heart of science, and must be built into medical education.

Close to questioning is controversy, and education – like newspapers – must encourage not suppress controversy. Because "When a thing ceases to be a subject of interest," said William Hazlitt, the British essayist, "it ceases to be a thing of interest." My final ingredient is creativity. "Imagination, "said Albert Einstein, the author of the theory of relativity, "is more important than knowledge."

So how does medical education stand up when measured against these criteria of mine: excitement, curiosity, awe, fun, stickability, questioning, controversy, and creativity? I leave readers to answer the question themselves, but I am not impressed.

What to read?

So if reading is as important as I've argued and if education should contain the ingredients I've suggested what should students be reading? Ultimately, my logic dictates, they must read whatever they want, but few students will resent guidance. I almost always will attempt to read a book or article recommended by a friend because if somebody is sufficiently inspired to recommend a piece of writing then there must be something worthwhile in the piece. Usually, that turns out to be right.

Textbooks are what medical students read most, and these are, I believe, what they should read least. Most textbooks are like frozen mammoths – dead and out of date. Worse, textbooks speak with a voice of authority when usually they are simply the world as it is temporarily agreed to be by a clutch of academics. They are uninteresting reading.

Much more interesting but also more difficult are the original articles that provide the intellectual base for medicine. Students cannot get all their knowledge from these papers, but learning to read them critically is a supremely important skill. Such reading will expose students to the fragility of medical knowledge and allow them to develop their humility, an essential feature in my mind of the good doctor. Learning to read these papers critically will also provide students with an essential tool for the whole of their professional life: they can then make informed assessments of all the many extravagant claims that will made to them by drug companies, governments, specialists, and a hundred and one other groups with vested interests.

There are articles that give advice on how to assess scientific papers critically (and they are all referenced in a paper by Fowkes and Fulton), and there are checklists that can be used for various different sorts of papers (see Table 1). But, as with most interesting activities, critical assessment cannot be reduced to a formula that can be used on all occasions because there are so many different sorts of papers. Furthermore, the way to develop the skill is to do it time and time again. It is also worth doing it with others, and journal clubs – where people present critical readings of papers – are useful learning devices. Students should also be helped to understand that they will not always get it "right" with a paper; medical journals regularly carry papers with important errors that the editors and reviewers have failed to spot.

Students should also be encouraged to read contemporary reviews – but again with a critical eye. Mulrow, Chalmers and others have pointed out that many reviews are very unscientific. The ideal reviewer frames a hypothesis, gathers together all relevant studies in all languages no matter whether published or unpublished, then sifts out all those that fall below a certain scientific standard, and combines those that remain. Rarely does this happen. More often the reviewer does a cursory search of familiar journals, skims the articles uncritically, mixes in his or her clinical prejudices, and writes the review. Students should be encouraged to assess reviews by going back to the original references; often they will discover that the original paper was scientifically unsound or concluded something quite different from what the reviewer said that it did.

Not just because I am the editor of one, I believe that students should be encouraged to read a general medical journal. They need to be exposed not only to the original articles and reviews that the journals contain but also to what I call the warp and woof of medicine – the politics, the controversies, the backbiting, the sociology, and the people. Students need to understand this wider world of medicine – and they will most likely enjoy it. Medical journals may often look boring, but they contain much that is interesting.

Something that is often found in medical journals that may be important for medical students to read are personal accounts of illness. Such accounts by doctors are published regularly in the BMJ, for instance, and the usual message is that there is an almost un-bridgeable gap between reading about a disease in a textbook or even treating patients with the disease and suffering from it. The insights that come from suffering from a disease almost always lead doctors to approach patients in a different way – at least at first. Students might also seek out literary accounts of illness: in them the quality of writing and insight will usually be higher than in a doctor's ac-count, but the author may have much broader aims than simply giving an account of his or her illness – and students must be cau-tious with their conclusions.

Few students find much time to read the history of medicine, but they would learn much if they did. They shouldn't read the history written by doctors which often present the progress of medicine as one breakthrough after another, but rather the history written by trained historians who point out the many blind alleys pursued by doctors – often at great expense in morbidity and mortality. They should not then fall into the trap of thinking that that was only yesterday and that now everything is smooth scientific progress. They might also read the English doctor Thomas McKeown's writings pointing out how deaths from infectious diseases had declined long before the organisms caus-ing them were identified and vaccines produced.

For the same reasons students should be exposed to some of the best writings criticising the quality of medical evidence – for instance, the writing of the American David Eddy and the Englis-hman Archie Cochrane's book "Effectiveness and efficiency". Also well worth reading are some of the polemical attacks on medicine – particularly that by the Austrian Ivan Illich who begins his book "limits to medicine" with the sentence: "The medical establishment has become a major threat to health." Students should encounter these books not to undermine their confidence in medicine but in order to develop the breadth essential for intellectual growth.

A further potentially rich area for study are comparisons among health care systems in different countries. These show how varied is the practice of medicine from country to country and how many different ways there are to organise health systems. It must be important as well for students to have some idea of how health care operates in developing countries: not only to make them aware of the effects of deep poverty but also to allow them to reflect how lessons learnt in developing countries are relevant in richer countries.

The reality of life for medical students is that they often have little time to read even the basic textbooks proffered to them by their teachers, but it would be a great shame if they never have time to read some of the great medically related novels – perhaps Middlemarch by George Eliot or The Citadel by A J Cronin – or some of the stories of Chekhov. There are also excellent accounts of medicine by outsiders – and one of the best of these is "A fortunate man" by the English writer John Berger.

This is an insightful account of the life of a country doctor in the Forest of Dean, a remote and poor area of England close to the border with Wales. Berger makes acute observations on the social position of the country doctor:

> He does more than treat them [his patients] when they are ill; he is the objective witness of their lives. They seldom refer to him as a witness. They only think of him when some practical circumstance brings them together. He is in no way a final arbiter. That is why I chose the rather humble word clerk: the clerk of their records.
>
> He is qualified to be this precisely because of his privilege. If the records are to be as complete as possible – and who does not at some times dream of the impossible ideal of being totally recorded? – the records must be related to the world at large, and they must include what is hidden, even what is hidden within the protagonists themselves.
>
> Some may now assume that he has taken over the role of the parish priest or vicar. Yet this is not so. He is not the representative of an all-knowing, all-powerful being. He is their own representative. His records will never be offered to any higher judge. He keeps the records so that, from time to time, they can consult them themselves. The most frequent opening to a conversation with him, if it is not a professional consultation, are the words 'Do you remember when...?'

Berger also observes how this country doctor, who commands huge respect, continues to learn:

His appetite for knowledge is insatiable. He believes that the limits of knowledge, at any given stage, are temporary. Endurance for him is no more than a form of experience, and experience is, by definition, reflective. It may be that in certain respects he is prepared to settle for comparatively little – for an obscure country practice, for a quiet domestic life, for a game of golf for relaxation. Within his outwardly circumscribed life, however, he is continually speculating about, extending and amending his awareness of what is possible. Partly this is the result of his theoretical reading of medicine, science, and history; partly it is the result of his own clinical observations. But above all it is the cumulative effect of his imaginative "proliferation" of himself in "becoming" one patient after another."

I quote this not only because it is a perceptive and attractive piece of writing about medicine by an outsider but also because it conveys something about how an "ordinary" doctor learns.

Finally, I think that medical students should read newspapers, not least because their patients read them. A constant danger for medical students is that there is such pressure on their time that they cease to pay attention to the larger world around them. This happened to me when I was a medical student – my "education" stopped me reading (and for the only time in my life) – but it is a sad thing that medical students should emerge from medical school less aware of the broader world than when they went in. (I'm struck by the prison style language that seems to come naturally.) But at the same time students shouldn't waste too much of their limited time on newspapers. Reading too many newspapers is like eating too much confectionery: students must also seek out good writing with its broader horizons. In the end, the best fiction is truer than newspapers.

I've developed here a guide to what students might read, but I believe passionately that students must be left to make their own journeys – otherwise, one of the major benefits of reading is lost. It was the American poet and physician Oliver Wendell Holmes who said: "The advice of their elders to young men is apt to be as unreal as the list of 100 best books."

How to read?

To obtain real benefit from reading students must be encouraged to read critically. Uncritical reading may positively mislead, although there may be times when really to appreciate fine writing it may be necessary to abandon yourself to the flow – like leaping from a plane. But to abandon yourself to a pulp novel is – in my elitist view – a waste. Life is too short to read rubbish, because it will never be possible to read all the truly good things worth reading. Thus I think that students should read broadly but wisely. It is important too that they read with engagement, excitement, pleasure, and a sense of discovery.

Writing

Medical journals are full of bad writing, and nobody caught this better than the British physician and writer, Richard Asher. In a memorable essay with the title "Why are medical journals so dull? he quoted a classic medical journal sentence:

> Experiments are described which demonstrate that in normal individuals the lowest concentration in which sucrose can be detected by means of gustation differ from the lowest concentration in which sucrose (in the amount employed) has to be ingested in order to produce a demonstrable decrease in olfactory acuity and a noteworthy conversion of sensations interpreted as satiety associated with ingestion of food.

Asher interpreted:

> Experiments are described which show that normal people can taste sugar in water in quantities not strong enough to interfere with their sense of smell or take away their appetite."

The causes of the writing that Asher parodies are slovenly thinking, laziness, and pomposity – a particular problem in medicine. The English writer George Orwell diagnosed the problem in an essay called "Politics and the English language".[14] It is essay worth reading time and time again not only because it is so perceptive in its diagnoses but also because it prescribes simple rules for putting the problem right. First his diagnosis:

> "As a man may take to drink because he feels himself to be a failure, and then fall more completely because he drinks. It is rather the same thing that is happening to the English language.

It becomes ugly and inaccurate because our thoughts are foolish, but the slovenliness of our language makes it easier for us to have foolish thoughts. The point is that the process is reversible. Modern English, especially written English, is full of bad habits which spread by imitation and which can be avoided if one is willing to take the necessary trouble. If one gets rid of these habits one can think more clearly, and to think more clearly is a necessary first step towards political regeneration: so that the fight against bad English is not frivolous and is not the exclusive concern of professional writers.

I do not read Norwegian or any other language, but I would be surprised if these comments were not applicable in all languages.

How to write better?

The difficult part of writing – particularly longer writing – is getting the structure right. No matter how beautifully the individual sentences are spun readers will grow exhausted if they have no sense of where the piece that they are reading is going. "Stream of consciousness" writing works only for superlative writers: the rest of us need to follow a clear structure. And if we do our pieces will be read even if the style is workaday. Because mostly people read medical writing not for the beauty or excitement of its style but rather for its content. Clarity is thus vital.

Structure may be best approached through questions. The English poet Rudyard Kipling wrote:

I keep six honest serving men
(They taught me all I knew);
Their names are What and Why and When
And How and Where and Who

The English medical statistician, Austin Bradford Hill, then adapted Kipling's idea to create the IMRAD structure, which is the form usually employed in medical journals. I stands for introduction, M for methods, R for results, and D for discussion, and each section of the paper is concerned with answering particular questions:

Introduction (Why you did it?)
Methods (What you did?)

Results (What you found?)
Discussion (What it means? What might be wrong? What next?)

There are several books on medical writing (15), and these elaborate on how to write medical papers using this structure. I don't want to elaborate any further on the topic here, but I have done so elsewhere (16).

But after getting the structure right the next task must be to spin the sentences. This should not be difficult so long as simple rules of brevity and clarity are kept in mind. Orwell – in the essay mentioned above – spelt out six rules for good writing:

1. Never use a metaphor, simile, or other figure of speech which you are used to seeing in print
2. Never use a long word where a short one will do
3. If it is possible to cut a word out, always cut it out
4. Never use the passive where you can use the active
5. Never use a foreign phrase, a scientific word or a jargon word if you can think of an everyday equivalent
6. Break any of these rules rather than say anything outright barbarous

Again I think that these rules should be applicable in any language.

Conclusion

You could probably be a doctor and never read, but, as Osler says, you'd not be much of one. To reach the wisdom, understanding, and breadth that, I believe, are essential for the great doctor broad reading is indispensable. Writing may be slightly less crucial, but even if they don't write for publication all doctors will have to write to patients, managers, and other doctors – and if they cannot write clearly and concisely they – and their patients – will suffer. Beyond straightforward communication writing will allow you to test out and organise your thinking, make discoveries, and enter the discourse that is essential for progress in medicine or in anything.

*Reproduced by permission of the authors and
the British Medical Journal*

Guidelines and checklist for appraising a medical article

Guideline	*Checklist*	
(1) Study design appropriate to objectives?	Objective:	Common design:
	Prevalence	Cross sectional
	Prognosis	Cohort
	Treatment	Controlled trial
	Cause	Cohort, case-control, cross sectional
(2) Study sample representative?	Source of sample	
	Sampling method	
	Sample size	
	Entry criteria/exclusions	
	Non-respondents	
(3) Control group acceptable?	Definition of controls	
	Source of controls	
	Marching/randomisation	
	Comparable characteristics	
(4) Quality of measurements and outcomes?	Validity	
	Reproducibility	
	Blindness	
	Quality control	
(5) Completeness?	Compliance	
	Drop outs	
	Deaths	
	Missing data	
(6) Distorting influences?	Extraneous treatments	
	Contamination	
	Changes over time	
	Confounding factors	
	Distortion reduced by analysis	

++ = Major problem.   0 = No problem.
 + = Minor problem.   NA = Not applicable.

References

1. Osler W. Aphorisms. Bean ED, ed. New York: Henry Schuman, New York, 1950: 124-5.
2. Borges JL. Labyrinths. Harmondsworth: Penguin, 1970.
3. Blishen E. The school that I'd like. Harmondsworth: Penguin, 1969.
4. Fraser RC. Undergraduate medical education: present state and future needs. BMJ 1991; 303: 41-3.
5. Fowkes FGR, Fulton PM. Critical appraisal of published research: introductory guidelines. BMJ 1991; 302: 1136-40.
6. Mulrow CD. The medical review article: state of the science. Ann Intern Med 1987; 104: 485-8.
7. Chalmers I. Improving the quality and dissemination of reviews of clinical research. In: Lock S, ed. The future medical journals. London: British Medical Journal, 1991.
8. McKeown T. The modern rise of population. London: Edward Arnold, 1976.
9. Eddy DM, Billings J. The quality of medical evidence: implications for quality of care. Health Affairs 1988 Spring; 19-32.
10. Cochrane A. Effectiveness and efficiency: random reflections on health services. London: Nuffield Provincial Hospitals Trust, 1971.
11. Illich I. Limits to medicine. London: Marion Boyars, 1976.
12. Berger J. A fortunate man. London: Allen Lane, 1967.
13. Asher R. Why are medical journals so dull? In: Asher R. A sense of Asher: a new miscellany. London: BMA, 1984.
14. Orwell G. Politics and the English language. In: Orwell G. The Penguin Essays of George Orwell. Harmondsworth: Penguin, 1984.
15. Lock S. Thorne's better medical writing. London: Pitman, 1977.
16. Smith R. How to get published. Practitioner 1987; 231: 961-7.
17. Smith R. Writing for medical journals. In: Gabbay J, ed. Guidelines on communication. London: Faculty of Public Health Medicine (in press).

The Conference Workshops

This section of the book is devoted to the workshops that formed the main part of the Oslo Conference programme. Chapter 10 describes their background, purposes, philosophy and methods, and then discusses their outcomes. It is suggested that workshops of this kind can provide participants with real opportunities to create their own conference to meet their own learning needs. Moreover, by allowing participants to propose their own workshop topics and to a large extent resource themselves, their emerging needs can be addressed as the conference proceeds.

A number of conclusions are drawn from this experience. Workshops can work at the level of individual participants, who seem to gain greatly in personal knowledge, but more tangible products are harder to achieve. The workshop process is difficult to capture.

Following this chapter, the workshop topics are listed, and the reports of them are printed as they appeared in the daily conference newspaper.

10

Workshops as Self-directed Adult Learning

COLIN COLES AND PHILIP BASHOOK

This chapter describes the background, purposes, philosophy and methods underpinning the workshops which formed a major element of the Oslo Conference and the outcomes of these workshops are reviewed. It is believed they fundamentally influenced the development of participants' personal knowledge, though it proved rather more difficult to produce detailed reports of the workshops themselves, so we list the workshop titles and print the brief reports that appeared each day in a conference newspaper.

Background

In planning the Oslo Conference it was quickly agreed that participants would gain most from it if they spent as much time as possible actively interacting with one another rather than sitting in a lecture room passively listening to speakers. Lectures, no matter how well intentioned, how expert their delivery, or how appropriate their message, were we felt not the best way to learn. Rather, the conference should strive to meet the demands made by, and opportunities afforded through, addressing the principles of adult learning. This seemed to suggest some kind of group work, possibly of a workshop nature.

It was recognised too by the planners that to do this would not be as simple as it sounded. The conference would bring together people from two quite distinct cultures – medicine and education. While we hoped this could provide the necessary conditions for positive and fruitful interaction, we also knew that these two groups had differing expectations of meetings and conferences, and that these differences could create tensions and conflicts which could be counterproductive.

All too frequently we have had the experience that when medical and educational people work together on common problems in medical education they can sometimes do so ineffectively, and we suspect that when this happens it is because, through pressures of time, they fail to share the fundamental assumptions they make from their intellectual and professional basis. Put another way, the "baggage" they have accumulated along their different ways is rarely "unpacked". As a result it seemed to us that medical and educational people tend to make inaccurate assumptions about, or fail to recognise, or just simply are totally ignorant of, what background knowledge and concepts in their own field inform what they say and do. People talk at cross purposes, and misunderstandings are all too common. This we felt would have serious implications here if we simply substituted workshops for the more commonly accepted lecture programme. We would after all be forcing people to sit and talk to each other for extended periods. We hoped they would speak the same language but we were not sure they would.

What are these differences that so concerned us? Medical people, we thought, tend to be task orientated. They like to intervene, to solve problems, to take action. They seem to prefer meetings with clearly defined events, so as to focus their efforts and not to waste time. There should be some tangible outcomes – something to take away and use. Meetings need to be relevant. Consensus should be achieved. Intellectual banter is all very well but in the end it's just a game.

Educationists, on the other hand, seemed to us to be more comfortable with an open agenda. They can rather more easily than medical people tolerate ambiguity. For them, learning can be equally valuable in the act of exploration as in the attainment of some goal. Indeed, some educators even seem to distrust goals, arguing "whose goal is it anyway?". For educators, the process can be more important than the product. Diversity of opinion is to be welcomed, even strived for.

While the educators who attended might be expected to accept a workshop approach and settle quickly to their task, medical people might need rather more persuasion, and this could apply even to those whose major interest is medical education.

In the pre-conference publicity, workshop topics were listed and participants were invited to make choices for the first two days. These topics were chosen to fit closely with the early keynote addresses, and to focus on topics thought to be of commonly agreed significance to participants as suggested by current trends in medical education. Following the early workshops, it was decided that participants themselves would create their own topics, and as far as possible lead and resource them. Early on, then, an element of choice was provided within a clear structure, and later on, as issues clarified or emerged through the conference, the workshop programme would become self generating. Put another way, the workshops as far as possible reflect the "learner-centred" approach we were taking to the conference as a whole.

Purposes

The workshops would serve a number of purposes. Fundamentally they would provide a practical demonstration of adult learning in a conference setting, that is they would give participants the opportunity for significant amounts of time during the meeting to reflect on their own experience, to recognise and articulate the personal knowledge on which they based their practice, and to come to see more clearly for themselves their own conceptualisations of problems and solutions in medical education.

The workshops would also provide participants from differing cultures, principally medicine and education, to share their perspectives and, at least in part, to appreciate, if not always clearly understand let alone entirely accept, the other person's point of view. There would be time for some kind of mutual intellectual exploration where each participant felt as safe and secure as possible, able to express doubts and uncertainties, or to try to put into words half considered viewpoints or conceptualisations.

Through the workshops we hoped people would generate understandings for themselves, to construct new knowledge, that would be of significance to them in their work, and with luck help them practise more effectively.

If possible, though by no means was this a requirement, participants might consider arriving at some consensual statements either in the course of their discussions or at their conclusion, and to prepare these in a form that could be shared with others either at a plenary session held at the end of the day, or through the conference newspaper which was printed every evening ready for the next day's breakfast table, or even to be written up for publication in this book. This gave us some concern though, and it is a concern voiced already: would the desire for some concrete outcome stultify the individual learning process? Our primary aim was that people would gain personal knowledge but we feared that any attempt to arrive at agreed conclusions could be counter-productive in achieving this. Striving for a group report could destroy the process of enlightenment for an individual. On the other hand, we also knew that the very act of attempting to summarise a conclusion could focus and even crystallise people's thoughts. We would have to be careful in requesting some tangible agreed product.

A final purpose was for workshops to create opportunities for people to build personal relationships in the context of medical education. One outcome that would be entirely satisfactory from the organisers' point of view would be for participants to meet others they didn't know before the conference took place, and to gain professionally through this contact. Perhaps as a bonus, people would stay in touch once the conference was over, to continue the sharing process and even work together again. The workshops could contribute to the all important "networking" we need for our practice. In a sense we hoped deliberately to create formally through the conference programme a way for networking to happen that sometimes emerges at more traditionally arranged meetings as a result of people's own efforts in their own time, at meals, or over a drink at the bar.

Philosophy

The philosophy behind the workshops was to be true to the principles of adult learning as we saw them. Personal choice has already been mentioned. So is the desire for participants to reflect on their experience, share their perspectives and to generate new personal knowledge. We felt too that people need to be responsible for defining their own learning objectives, not "out of the blue", nor without consideration of the range of alternatives, nor without hearing and possibly accepting what others think they ought to be learning, but through informed choice and by being helped to reflect on their practice.

People should have the chance to attempt to achieve their learning objectives through their own efforts, and by cooperation and collaboration with others, accepting and acknowledging the resources provided by other people's experience and expertise. We felt we should provide as nearly as possible the optimal conditions for effective learning, not the competitive and combative ones sometimes seen in medical education. Moreover, we felt people should apply and further develop their skills of evaluating their own progress in achieving their objectives, and through interaction with others find new ways of achieving their goals.

As a consequence, we hoped people would perceive new gaps in their knowledge and experience, and demand further opportunities to meet these needs as the conference proceeded.

Methods

To achieve all of this we recognised that we had to provide certain resources. Adequate time was needed for the workshops to work. Participants would need to establish effective working methods. The basic group processes of forming, storming, norming and performing would need to be activated as quickly as possible. Even so these group processes themselves would take time. We allowed from 9.30 am to 4.30 for workshops to operate. In this way, we felt enough time was available for discussions to develop. People would be given sufficient scope within reasonable time limits.

When each workshop convened, the process began with brief introductions. Participants discussed ideas and issues they hoped would be considered during the workshop session. Most workshops used a nominal group process with workshop moderators serving as group process facilitators and in some instances preparing verbal and written reports. The workshop participants were expected to explore topics in as much depth and breadth as participants desired. All the workshops were designed to employ adult learning principles and foster self-directed learning at a pace and intensity that participants found mutually acceptable.

Next, the environment needed to be conducive to working in this way. The conference venue, Soria Moria, provides just the right conditions. There are enough rooms of the right size to accommodate groups ranging from five to twenty people at a time. The rooms are furnished with comfortable chairs around tables that can be moved to any configuration the participants felt was useful. Rooms have marker boards and flip charts, and could use overhead projectors or video recorders if needed.

Each group had a facilitator to lead them who had some previous experience of this role and knew what was needed. In particular they recognised their task was to encourage discussion and to involve everyone, yet to provide some focus and framework to keep those discussions "on track". Groups also needed someone with particular experience or knowledge to act as a resource. This meant identifying people who had something to offer, some contribution to make that was relevant to the topic but who would only provide this expertise as and when it was needed, that is when the participants wanted it or the facilitator judged the time right for this to happen. This was pre-arranged for the early workshops. As the conference proceeded the organisers were gratified, and to some extent relieved, that facilitators and resource people "emerged" from amongst the participants themselves. The workshops truly became self generating and self resourced.

Daily verbal briefings of workshop happenings and the presentation of the products of the day's work were held in the late afternoon. This was also the opportunity to "advertise" the next day's workshops, and for potential workshop leaders to recruit participants. Both the initial workshops and those generated by participants' interests during the conference were chronicled in the daily conference newspaper.

Outcomes

Did the workshops work? How far did they achieve their purposes? At one level they clearly worked. Workshops were held, new topics were proposed, people attended, plenary reports were made, and daily newspaper copy was filed. Individual participants commented that they had achieved a great deal from the workshop process. A post-conference evaluation generated comments such as "Every workshop I participated in opened my mind, and new angles to problems developed", "Workshops provided the opportunity for standing back and reflecting, rather than leaping in to fill knowledge gaps", "The workshops were very important because they were quite 'allowing'", "It was fun to create something, to be creative and productive in regard to my own work".

Certainly too the workshops contributed to the life of the conference itself. They generated an enthusiasm for working, and gave a "buzz" to meal breaks and social events. It was quite common to hear people telling others what they had been doing in their particular workshop. Some topics were repeated on subsequent days because they had gained a reputation for being highly relevant for those who had missed them first time round.

Workshops also lead to the modification of the conference programme. Subsequent keynote addresses drew on the experience of the workshops and referred to the workshop reports groups made in the newspapers. An additional address was included since the topic proposed – medical education in an East European country – was seen to be potentially of value to all rather than offering it as a choice for a few.

If participants gained personal knowledge and the conference itself grew as a result of the workshop programme, what of the more tangible products? Three workshop reports were offered as contributions to this book which represented the output of groups where the participants or the facilitator felt a need to write down and share more widely the elements of their discussion. They were not extensive. Indeed they were rather brief reports. They were not richly referenced. They by no means exhaustively "covered" the topic. Yet they attempted to indicate honestly the thinking going on in the groups, and provided examples of how professionals meeting together under the conditions outlined above are able to challenge existing ideas, question previously held positions, and generate ideas that were new at least for themselves.

These contributions were considered very carefully in the process of editing this book. In the end they have not been included, not because the ideas were irrelevant, nor because the thoughts expressed were unworthy. Nor even was it thought that others would gain nothing from considering them. Rather, they have been omitted on two counts. First we felt the reports were unable to capture the workshop processes. The writers were too concerned with what was said rather than why or how it was said. Second the content of the reports looked frankly inchoate after the event. It seems that listing the outcomes of a group cannot capture the essence of what links those items together in people's minds. Knowledge of this kind is not only personal, it is always provisional. Writing about it objectively loses its essential subjectivity.

Conclusions

What have we learnt from the experience of running these workshops in this way as a significant aspect of such a conference? We are convinced that they achieved their main purpose of providing opportunities for personal growth. Participants told us that the workshops had lead them to meaningful learning which they felt they could apply in their own professional practice. Their tacit knowledge had developed, for some extensively, as a result. Some now felt able to explicate ideas they had long held dear but which until then they had appreciated only dimly. We are convinced too that producing "hard copy" from workshops is an unenviable task. Certainly it has eluded us on this occasion. Perhaps we expected too much. Perhaps we do not yet have the skills to capture the essence of workshops in a form that can be reproduced and published in a form which others, who inevitably are outsiders to that process, can benefit. Perhaps it is not even a worthwhile endeavour to pursue. Were we right all along in our belief that the attempt to arrive at consensual statements can inhibit the personal growth of individuals?

What then do we consider we would need to do at future workshops to get closer to producing helpful reports? We suggest three minimal conditions based on our experience here:

First, workshop groups would need to contain trained observers, who would do much more than record events or even act as a group secretary. They should not be contributors to the group process but should, like an anthropologist, observe the various interactions going on, people's affect, the ebb and flow of the discussion, the pace, etc. They should be skilled at picking up nuances, and recording critical incidents.

Second, workshop participants should discuss whether or not they want there to be some product from their session. Such a decision should not be taken lightly, and should be sensitively facilitated. People should know why they are being asked the question, and consider carefully what it might mean to agree or not. Above all they should debate what the consequences might be for their own personal growth. And the workshop organisers should be prepared for the group to reject the offer.

Third, immediately after the workshop the observer should informally interview participants, summarise the observations, write the report, and discuss it with the facilitator and key resource people who had been involved in the group work.

For the present, the products of our workshops are best seen in what we tried to do, how we did it, and our reflections on what happened. The list of workshop titles and the reports as they appeared in the daily news sheets are the tangible evidence of the workshops' success, and are reprinted next. Less objective yet clearly highly significant is the personal development of the workshop participants and the undoubted growth in their tacit knowledge and understanding. In the end, this may well be what learning is all about.

Workshop topics

Workshops were organised on the following topics.

1. Self-directed Lifelong Learning
   Moderators: Penny Jennett (Canada) and Philip Bashook (USA)
2. Modes of Thinking of Medicine, Teaching and Learning
   Moderators: Gunnar Handal, Per Lauvås, Kirsten Hofgaard
   Lycke (Norway)
3. Patient Education
   Moderator: Colin Coles (UK)
4. The Role of the Medical Educator
   Moderator: Dick Mårtenson (Sweden)
5. Problem-based Learning
   Moderator: Dick Mårtenson (Sweden)
6. Managing Change in a Medical Context
   Moderator: Janet Grant (UK)
7. Coping with Chronic Disease
   Moderators: Kent R. Montin and Karin Wikblad (Sweden)
8. Knowledge-based Decision Support as a Vehicle for Opportunistic Learning
   Moderators: Peter Pritchard (UK) and Ola Lilleholt (Norway)
9. Medical Audit – an Effective Method in Continuing Medical Education
   Moderators: Bjørn Oscar Hoftvedt and Sverre Lundevall (Norway)
10. Educating the Educators
    Moderators: Kirsten Hofgaard Lycke (Norway), Philip Bashook (USA), Colin Coles (UK)
11. Stimulating Students to become Change Agents/Students as Educators
    Moderator: Guttorm Brattebø (Norway)
12. Constructing a Learning Contract
    Moderator: Dick Mårtenson (Sweden)

Daily conference newspaper

A conference newspaper was produced daily which reported on the ideas and thoughts generated during workshops. These reports were typed up by workshop participants and printed overnight. They are presented here unedited, exactly as they appeared next morning for conference participants to read at breakfast.

1. Self-directed lifelong learning

Moderators: Phil Bashook, Penny Jennett

We approached the task of our group by attempting to define what we wished to call self-directed learning. In the process we focused mostly on the medical school context and reflected upon how the medical school training could contribute to lifelong learning in residency and practice.

We defined three foci for our discussions and explored in some depth each issue.

I.   What is self-directed learning, lifelong learning?
II.   Why is it critical
III. What is the best way to implement it?

I. What is self-directed learning?

It is continuous renewal of knowledge, methods, and craft as a result of professional experience. Included in this renewal process are the following components: taking responsibility for your own competence (learning); self-initiation and continuing curiosity, using trial and error; reaching out for challenges; getting essential information; having opportunity for needed reflection; working in a climate of openness with critical analysis but free from an external negative judgmental atmosphere. As a result of self-directed learning one displays spontaneously an expertise using intuition and one's art of medical practice. With greater expertise the process shifts from self-awareness to automatic functioning.

II. Why is it critical?

During professional practice self-directed learning comes from testing your competence against reality (success/failure). This process may lead to a need for correction and/or to supplement knowledge or skills fuelled by ambitions or curiosity and inhibited by rigidity, mindlessness or exhaustion. The undergraduate study could be/should be a model learning environment/process that fosters self-directed learning. Two sources of feedback suggesting further learning are: complaints from patients about professional behaviour (communication/information); medical misadventures identified by peers (out-of-date, referral omission). Self-directed learning is inspired by an enquiring mind, comfortable recognition of your professional limits, responding positively to the element of surprise, adjusting to deviations and variations from the norm, which triggers renewal of knowledge.

III. What is the best way to implement it?

There are three elements to implementing a self-directed learning process: knowledge, attitudes and skills. One needs to recognise the need to acquire and to maintain professional competence. Also, one should identify the tools and resources required (teachers, patients, colleagues, equipment and learning technology), and develop the skills and abilities to use them. Above all one must value the habit of self-directed learning. Several factors can enhance implementing self-directed learning. These are: experience, anchor points, comfort, responsibility, reflection, enthusiasm, reason for learning, openness, multi-professional learning, and learning in groups. Barriers to implementation include: reduced scheduled time (alternative is increased free time), reduce lecture hours and passive learning (promote active and independent learning, e.g. problem solving), use multiple resources, focus on the process rather and less on the content, shift responsibility from the teacher to the student, greater emphasis on evaluating the ability for self-learning and less on knowledge.

2. Modes of thinking in medicine. Teaching and learning

Moderators: Gunnar Handal, Per Lauvås, Kirsten Hofgaard Lycke

The moderators led with a presentation of Jürgen Habermas' analysis of rationality. He described three kinds:

1. Technical rationality (means/ends), orientated towards results.
2. Communicative rationality, orientated towards understanding.
3. Critical rationality, orientated towards validity.

The group were then presented with case material, with the suggestion that they write down and discuss how they would *act*, and how they *thought* they made the decision.

People's responses did not all conform to Habermas' analysis, and some participants resisted its application in the clinical setting. This led to contradictions, which were resolved by the moderators' decision to have an open agenda for the afternoon session.

This started with an impromptu presentation of Janet Grant's major research work on describing the thinking processes of medical students and doctors, and the changes as one matured into the other. She described three important findings.

1. The *process* of thinking is the same for students and experienced clinicians. Only the *content* was different.
2. The memory structure defines how people use knowledge – both the way it is stored and what is stored. The size of the memory store is the same for students and clinicians.
3. The "way out of a problem" depends on the identification of "forceful features". These were different for different individuals. The difference between student and expert lay in the expert's more effective and appropriate access to better – organised knowledge. She mentioned the development of a "diagnostic thinking inventory" of 35 items, currently being validated.

Kent Montin described his work on conceptualising medical science, in particular in the content of the diabetic care team. He quoted Aaron Antonovsky's work on "sense of coherence".

Gunnar Handal related the rationality to the role of the teacher. General discussion followed, with Anna-Karin Furhoff commenting that this was a "safe" group in which to describe one's thinking.

The group was open and participative, with a final comment that overcoming the earlier contradiction was a measure of the success of this productive group.

3. Patient education

Moderator: Colin Coles

We started with analyzing what patient education could be and the group suggested the following:

- helping/supporting the patients to learn
- learning from the patients
- changing attitudes
- counselling
- educating the general public
- educating relatives/families
- being patient while educating

We discussed some problem areas in relation to patient education and ended up with a long list. Here are some of the areas:

- perceived and expected roles and attitudes of health workers and patients.
- who defines health, illness and disease?
- how should "patient education" be labelled: consultation, check-up, meeting, appointment or education?
- how is the patient looked upon; as an object or a subject, as a grown-up or a child?
- how could or should we avoid moralistic attitudes towards patients with e.g. obesity, smoking problems.
- how do we know when a person has been "educated"? Is it when he is able to cope with his problems or is it when he has become a compliant patient?
- who decides the criteria for goal achievement?

We listed five questions we wanted to discuss:

1. What should health workers know about patient education?
2. How can the health care system adapt to become patientcentred?
3. What is preventing patient-centred education from happening?
4. How might patient-centred education be introduced?
5. How would we know if it is working?

We concentrated our discussion on questions no. 1 and 3.

Question 1. What should health workers know basically about patient education?

- *Start* where the patient is concerning
  * knowledge
  * beliefs and misbeliefs
  * social context and life situation
  * goals and ambitions
  * sources of knowledge
  * psychological state, etc.

- *How* to start where the patient is:
  * observing
  * asking open questions
  * listening

* avoiding too early "closure"
* using the patient's common sense
* using appropriate language
* help the patient to define learning objectives
* allow the patient to be active in the learning process

- Education is more than telling people things; it is about knowing, understanding and acting based on a choice.

Question 3. What is preventing patient-centred education from happening?

- Perceived roles and expectations in both health workers and patients. For example, the physician views himself as an expert, authority and might be disease-centred. The patient takes the passive role.

Health care system-centred philosophy dominates over patient-centred philosophy.

4. The role of the medical educator

Moderator: Dick Mårtenson

What is a (medical) educator? A broad definition could be:
Any person responsible for conveying medical knowledge, skills and attitudes to others.
Definition in functional terms:

* conveys a message (communicates in a wide sense)
* facilitates a learning process
* is an expert in some field
* is open minded
* cares about students (patients.)
* is enthusiastic
* engages in a two-way process

We discussed educators on different levels of the education system, and that students also should function as educators.
When creating a climate that stimulates sound learning, the medical educator and the system must:

1) be open to innovation and be flexible
2) stimulate the joy, and motivation for learning – encourage curiosity, teach values, caring, ethics
3) encourage cooperation and not competition
4) integrate teaching, research and practice
5) integrate the phases of lifelong learning across the stages of undergraduate training > postgraduate training > continuous education (e.g. a planned and coordinated curriculum as for drug abuse/alcohol)
6) give regular feed-back to the doctor/student (standards of knowledge and practice)
7) handle information overload – assist in sorting out

How to stimulate good learning approaches among students?
The assessment procedures have a strong impact on what and how students learn!

Basically it is more an issue of students' attitudes towards learning approaches than specific study-skills or behaviours. What ought to be achieved in any curriculum is to make students aware of the phenomena.

Encourage students to be critical of authorities, to frequently ask "what is the evidence of this?" and "why is it so?".

The meaning of the term "knowledge" must be reflected upon by students and trainees (from 'is in a textbook' to 'is applicable to clinical situations' to 'is internalised').

Prepare undergraduate students that good learning-approaches sometimes are difficult to use under working conditions.

Study-approaches are an integral part of PBL.

Should one force students into learning approaches they are unfamiliar with or that they a priori dislike? There are arguments for and against.

5. Problem-based learning

Moderator: Dick Mårtenson

WHAT IS PROBLEM-BASED LEARNING ?
PBL is agreed upon to be a strategy to design objectives,teaching/ learning activities, content and evaluation beginning with problems, in our case health problems.

EVOLUTION OF LEARNING IN MEDICINE
- apprenticeship
- discipline-based curriculum (independent, dependent, integrated)
- competence-based curriculum
- problem-based curriculum

WHY CHANGE ?
1. relative concerns:
   - to increase the ability to use knowledge
   - to increase relevance (of contents, etc.)
   - to increase the ability to solve new problems
   - to motivate students by – exposure to real life problems – social obligation to peers
   - to motivate to work as a team
   - to increase the ability to communicate
   - to avoid "coveritis" (a curriculum disease tending to swallow all time)
   - to increase and motivate to learn in a self-directed way by – flexibility in time – facilitating resource use
   - to make it more enjoyable (challenging but not easier!!!)
   - to increase retention of memory
   - to improve learning approaches
2. educational theory results
3. research results in physiology

HOW TO DO IT?
After getting case reports from Linkøping, Tromsø and Bahrain we refined the following essentials of problem-based learning in practice appreciating differences in planning, organisation and implementation:

- diminish the power of departments/increasing the power of study committees
- integration in terms of organ systems
- written health problems
- self-directed learning
- small group tutorials/tutor training
- early clinical exposure
- increase in unscheduled time
- early identification as doctor

We would like to propose the following strategy:

Adapt the general principles to the specific circumstances – do not copy!!!

6. Managing change in medical context

Moderator: Janet Grant

The entire workshop consisted of a set of exercises, with plenary discussions in between on general aspects that derived from the participants' experiences of those exercises. Individually and in groups of increasing size good and bad aspects of change management were identified. In another exercise learning needs of the participants' were brought through small group tutorials. In one exercise a case was presented. The scenario was about the process of implementing a change for career counselling and monitoring for junior doctors at the fictitious Grimstoke Hospital.

The entire day was mind-blowing! Hence a brief summary will not be just to the quality of the discussions made.

Most of the good and bad aspects agreed upon, could be regarded as being on a continuum, or given positive/negative connotations depending on what frame of reference you use when judging. Some of the aspects identified were:

Good	**Bad**
Challenge;	Creates new
excitement;	problems; time
freshness;	consuming; causes
rejuvenating;	conflicts.
individual	
satisfaction and	Uncertainty;
interpersonal	losses; survival.
relationship;	
stimulate	Painful to change
activities.	(though if there
	is a need to
Reflection;	change there must
broadened	be a pain in
perspectives.	the system)
Possible	
(not unrealistic)	
improvements.	

A remark on learning needs: Important for non-medical change agents to get close to the medical culture, i.e. experiencing it, trying to understand it.

Two conclusions to emphasize:

Very important for a change-agent to be careful in facilitating the identification of the true nature of the problem, and to ascertain that the clients have a shared and joint perception of the problem/s. That part of the change process must have sufficient time.

In planning a change process, concentrate carefully on the opposing factors, the perceived obstacles. Forces for a change will likely remain, forces against must be, if possible, foreseen and then taken care of (which takes time and could slow down the pace).

7. Coping with a chronic disease

Moderators: Kent Montin and Karin Wikblad

The workshop started with a short description of coping based on the Sense of Coherence theory. The question then discussed was: "Why do some patients cope well while others do not"? There are no good or bad coping strategies in patients with chronic diseases but instead complete or incomplete strategies which means the level at which a patient can develop and maintain biological, psychological and social balance.

Coping as seen from the patient's perspective may be different from the perspective of health professionals. To unite possibly divergent views it is important to create a climate where the patient is capable of asking the relevant questions and can answer them. The problems inherent in coping with chronic disease seen from different perspectives may be illustrated in the graphic model below.

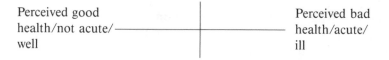

Pathology/severity/disease

| Perceived good health/not acute/ well | | Perceived bad health/acute/ ill |

No pathology/lack of severity/no disease

A traditional medical orientation moves up and down along the vertical axis. A patient will move back and forth on the horizontal axis. The position of the patient at any given time could be anywhere in the four quadrants, not necessarily mutually congruent as seen from the patient and the doctor.

Example: A diabetic may perceive good health and place himself/herself in the bottom left corner quadrant, while the doctor recognising the patient as a heavy smoker and having hypertension will place the patient in the upper left quadrant. The patient feels that he/she is coping well; should the doctor induce him/her to change the coping strategy. The answer may be yes or no.

The model was tested for medical implications in a variety of chronic diseases and acute illness, even mental disorder, and was found applicable.

Remaining problems for discussion were:

1. Educational diagnosis or assessment: How should physicians and other health personnel deal with this? How should the curriculum be arranged to prepare health personnel for this? How should health personnel be trained for this?
2. Media give out misleading or too optimistic information about cures and hopes for patients with a chronic disease, leading to disruption of on-going strategies, creating problems both for them and the care-teams.

These could be topics for another workshop.

8. Knowledge-based decision support and opportunistic learning

Moderators: Peter Pritchard and Ola Lilleholt

The general theme of the workshop was the future impact that new and advanced information technology might have on the practice and learning of medicine.

A "hypertext"-based system developed by Dr Ola Lilleholt was demonstrated, and then the "Oxford System of Medicine", under development at the Imperial Cancer Research Fund was described. The workshop then worked in groups, and discussed the benefits and adverse effects of advanced information technology in the context of each participant's work. The following comments were made.

Beneficial effects	Adverse effects
Safe decisions	Divert GP's attention from patient's need
Memory jogger	Reduce contact with colleagues
Quicker update of knowledge	Technology displaces humanity and social context
Better quality assurance	Overlooking non-verbal communication
Administrative efficiency (daily routines)	Reducing drive to remember and structure, knowledge and thinking
Teaching information search	Upset existing habits

In the second session, there was a presentation on the gap between knowledge held by specialists and patients. The patient was also cast in the role of an expert. The general practitioner was seen to have a bridging role in transferring knowledge between specialist and patient and vice versa. Lay self-help groups might have a bridging role too, and it was seen as important that GPs should share knowledge with them. Such groups might have a particular function in helping patients to explicate their health beliefs. Knowledge-based systems were effective at the GP–specialist knowledge interface, but ineffective, at present, at the GP–patient interface.

There followed an active discussion of the nature of medical knowledge and the effects that knowledge-based systems might have on continuing medical education, but no firm conclusions were reached. The future of textbooks and journals was discussed, and their future niche seemed assured.

The workshop covered a broad range of topics and the need for emphasis on the human aspects of new technology was stressed. This would have major implications for education.

9. Medical audit – peer review – effective methods in continuing medical education

Moderators: Björn Oscar Hoftvedt and Sverre Lundevall

Peer review groups are used in general practice for a variety of purposes. The most common purpose is to identify needs for CME and as a tool for quality assurance. As a spin-off the participants also get a deeper knowledge of the character of their practice and perhaps of general practice as such.

We heard accounts of three types of peer review in general practice. The groups consisted of six to eight GPs with a moderator. The first group discussed their referrals of patients to hospital departments, the second random consultations from the practice and the third patients with a specific symptom or disease.

It was obvious that the participants in all three groups found the work enjoyable and useful, although it was not always easy to pinpoint in what way.

In our analysis of the three types of peer review we reached the conclusion that peer review could be seen as consisting of two stages.

In the first stage, the group discussed single cases, preferably with a leader and using some kind of standardised format. This would help the GP to manage the patient under discussion in a more efficient way, and could also identify some needs for CME. It also gave the satisfaction of knowing that you were not the only one having problems in the management of patients – it is a great help to share your insecurity with others.

In the second stage, the material discussed (the randomly selected consultations, the patients with a certain symptom, the referrals) was put together and statistically analyzed. Several important things could be gained by this.

- the doctor would be able to know his/her own profile compared to the group as a whole, concerning type of patients, types of diagnoses, prescription habits, etc., which would provide a much more valid basis for CME than the discussion of single cases, and which could also be used as indicators of quality,
- this combined view of the practice of several GPs could generate hypotheses, which could be tested, and which could constitute a starting-point for a scientific approach to general practice.

Factors supporting peer review

Peer review is important in Norway where participating in a peer review group is a recognised way of GP's meeting CME recertification requirements. This has several advantages. There are trained (and paid!) leaders, and these leaders can be supported in their turn. There is a structure which can make the work easier for the participants, and also facilitate the statistical analysis. A feeling of mutual basic trust among the group members is a prerequisite.

Access to computers will facilitate the statistical analysis. Indeed, if the practice records are computerised, peer review could start directly at the second stage.

Barriers to peer review

In most countries, lack of time would be the greatest barrier to peer review. Fear of exposure is a real hindrance for many. Doubts about the effectiveness of peer review as an instrument of CME, and the difficulty to prove its worth, are other negative factors.

10. Teaching teachers to teach

Moderators: Kirsten Hofgaard Lycke, Philip Bashook, Colin Coles

It was agreed that the main question to be addressed in this workshop was "how best can we replicate medical educators?" To do this, participants began by telling their own stories concerning their personal professional development. They were encouraged to identify key, pivotal times in their careers which particularly looked at what point they felt comfortable doing what they do. In this way people might convey ideas through their stories. Inevitably these stories were anecdotal and autobiographical. It became clear that people had quite differing experiences, on widely varying timescales, and many of the "key" moments had only taken on significance as a consequence of the reflection they had just been asked to perform. Despite this variability certain common features could be identified. Personal experience was a crucial basis for subsequent significant insight. Often this seemed to result from "theoretical" study of abstract principles after rather than before these experiences. This helped the person to make sense of, or account for, aspects of their experience.

From these "stories" participants began to build models. In this phase of the workshop, people agreed to adhere to two ground rules: first, not to engage too early in "closure" and second not to reject a previously suggested model but to build on what had gone before in a collaborative and constructive manner.

Two major contributions were formulated by way of model building. One looked at the possible tensions between the apparently distinct cultures or communities of education and medicine. Defining characteristics were discussed, in particular, noting that while the culture of medicine included the practice of education, the culture of education did not include the practice of medicine. An interesting discussion focused on the place of "health education" taught in schools. Was this an exception where medicine was practised within education? The general feeling was that while medicine "informed" health education, it was not medicine that was being practised. Indeed, it was noted that school-based health education tended to be undervalued by the medical profession.

Participants discussed what it meant for a practitioner in one culture or the other to move across cultures. Clearly there are implications for both doctors and educators. One implication is the process of becoming socialised into the new culture. Another was the need for an organisational structure that can incorporate these individuals into the professional community. In some settings (for example, in the USA) there is a critical mass of individuals forming a new culture/community which is being called "Medical Education". Two necessary ingredients are individuals who have developed the expertise to be medical educators, and the creation of position for them.

A second model was proposed to help explain how new medical educators could be produced, and was termed "Lego" (after the child's constructional toy). This has three features: pictures on the box (which equates with concrete experiences), pieces inside the box (or abstract principles on which we base practice), and seeing one's task as piecing together the pieces to make something which replicates the picture (which is what the medical educator does).

The workshop concluded by defining some key attributes of medical educators:

- working in a functional orientation
- being product orientated
- being a risk taker
- being enthusiastic
- having the ability to define "pictures", "pieces", and "tasks"
- being confident enough in your own discipline to be able to let go of it
- knowing what you can do and what you can't do
- valuing and respecting the profession of medicine as it exists rather than wanting to change it

11. Stimulating students to become change agents and students as educators

Moderator: Guttorm Brattebø

We defined the targets for our discussion to be "What can be done in order to stimulate students to become change agents in so called traditional curricula where improvements are badly needed?" and "General aspects to be considered when using students as instructors".

To the issue of change agents we concluded that it is a neglected area, because most efforts so far have been directed towards increasing the pedagogical competence of teachers. The following domains were discussed:

- Students need to be informed of the formal and informal channels as well as "rules of the game" within an institution from the very beginning of their medical studies.
- Potential of change: in a small school it is assumed that it is easier to change (despite the fact that there are small schools with very minor improvements), and that in a large school it is almost impossible due to the large number of students. In principle the potential ought to be higher in large schools because "big is strong".
- Impeding factors: students' ignorance of educational principles and alternatives; inter-student relations (the lonely wolf & who cares vs solidarity and caring for student fellows); cultural factors like relation of teachers-students (authoritarianism) or the acceptance of criticism.
- It is important to consider the institutional context and educational climate. In an environment with some well-designed courses, or with some decent assessments, the strategies would differ from a medical school lacking positive examples. Local regulations and political or organisational aspects must be regarded.
- Strategies: Any strategy will depend on local conditions. We discussed only in general terms and emphasised that (a) it is important to increase the students' awareness of vital pedagogical issues including their roles in developing their learning environment, (b) next step would be defining and sharing a central problem to attack, (c) maybe collecting data, (c) ensure visibility and present in a convincing manner, (d) not being afraid of taking calculated risks and confrontations, (e) to a greater extent use existing student-networks and share concrete examples of alternative learning modes in use.

It was proposed that a booklet ought to be written. The booklet should provide examples of successful events promoting students' willingness to constructively change. For instance the so called "survival and guerilla" workshop recently held in Tromsö, the student strike in Berlin, student activities at Karolinska, meaningful in-course evaluations, etc. The booklet should also elaborate on principles raised in the workshop Managing change in medical context.

There are several good reasons and experiences from having older students function as educators for younger students: older students being tutors in problem-based tutorials at Herdecke, the mixed groups at Kansas City in Missouri, students acting as leaders of colloquia, etc. A student should though not be put in the task of providing lectures.

12. Constructing a learning contract

Moderator: Dick Mårtenson

Learning contracts have been used i CME and post-graduate training, though not in undergraduate programmes. The main conclusions from the workshop were:

The device "contract learning" does not seem irrelevant, it makes sense. It seems to be feasible to construct meaningful items in a contract.

The group started by identifying the following "domains" to discuss and used one hour to clarify them in sub-groups:

Reasons for using contract learning. Preconditions to be met for a contract: (a) a mutual interest between partners, i.e. goals, (b) can be defined or negotiable, (c) both partners responsible for fulfilling the contract. Reasons for using it: (i) clarifies and visualises the responsibilities between the contractors, (ii) creates a good and safe learning climate, (iii) a tool for mutual feed-back, (iv) secures justice in use of educational resources.

What parties and persons could be included in a contract? Teacher – student/s; GP – student/s; curriculum committee – department/course; student/s – nurses; the student him-/herself (a signed contract with oneself).

Content in a contract: we identified headings like WHAT (knowledge, skills, attitudes as can be found in any syllabus; behaviours; expected activities and contributions; personal aspects like empathy, ability to listen, timekeeping, being prepared; process-factors like those stated for PBL-tutorials. HOW covering all practical means like the use of different sources for learning, feed-back sessions, assignments, etc. The WHEN and ASSESSMENT PROCEDURES. We did not discuss, though arrived several times at the issues of, what will happen and how to handle situations when contracts are not met, as well as what basic attitudes do those who create the contracts have?

Conclusions

This chapter brings together the major features of this book. It begins by describing the traditional approach to medical education and discusses its inherent weaknesses. Then, drawing on the various ideas and experiences expressed throughout the book, it shows the progress being made in contemporary medical educational practice towards a more enlightened approach. The chapter then examines some recent educational theories far removed from medical education itself in an attempt to explain why the traditional approach fails to provide more appropriate education yet the contemporary approach apparently succeeds. On this basis it proposes a theory for medical education, and challenges teachers, learners, and institutions to face their own unique responsibilities.

11

Learning in Medicine: Towards a Theory of Medical Education

COLIN COLES AND HANS ASBJØRN HOLM

The traditional approach

Traditional medical education is largely concerned with "pot filling" (1), that is by teachers passing on information to learners. It is personified by the lecture, which sometimes is described as the transmission of information from the lecturer's notes to the student's notes, without passing through the minds of either! Teaching is telling. The teacher is active, the learner is passive.

Very typically, too, medical education is often separate from the practice of medicine. In the undergraduate medical curriculum the pre-clinical course is often separated from the clinical course, and the basic sciences are often located separately from the wards. What is more, theory is usually presented prior to its application. The firmly held belief is that students must learn what are often called "the basics" before they are able to apply them. Even in postgraduate medical education, teaching is frequently separated from practice. If doctors want to learn something new, or if they must prepare for some examination, they attend a course, or apply for study leave. Much of their formalised education is "off-the-job".

Even where postgraduate and continuing medical education are not separated from practice, that is when it is actually "on-the-job" education, the traditional approach is for senior medical staff to tell their juniors what they are doing wrong and what they should be doing. There is very little feedback to the learners on their performance, and even when it is given it is frequently negative.

Often traditional medical education is authoritarian. The teachers are in charge. They are the people who know. The learners are those who do not know. The teacher's job is therefore to pass on knowledge. Medical Education is also hierarchic. The teacher is superior to the learner. There is a high degree of control. Examinations for example provide a means whereby the trainee is allowed entry into the profession or to a particular medical specialty. They are rites of passage. Medical education means learners overcoming successive hurdles. Examinations judge people's performance, and even punish the weak. They rarely provide feedback for learners to understand where they are going wrong and what they need to do in order to improve. Medical education is coercive too. There is nothing other than for trainees to endure the privations imposed by it. In many ways it is paternalistic. It is a parent–child relationship (2) rather than a meeting of equals.

Weaknesses of the traditional approach

The traditional approach to medical education has a number of consequences (3,4,5). Frequently, people who are experiencing difficulties with their education describe feeling overloaded with content. There is so much to do, and so little time in which to do it. They experience a loss of motivation. People enter medicine with a high degree of commitment, often this dissipates during their education. Some researchers describe a corresponding increase in people's cynicism and a decreased ability to show empathy (6). The pre-clinical and clinical courses are sometimes dubbed the pre-cynical and cynical!

Traditional medical education leads to a deterioration of people's approaches to studying (7). Whereas students enter medical school with apparently desirable ways of studying, these quickly deteriorate as the course proceeds. Rather than trying to understand the meaning of what one is learning, students quickly realise that what they need to do is to rote learn lists of facts in order to pass the next examination in a parrot-like fashion. They quickly forget what they have learnt and fail to apply much of it in a practical setting (8).

With the overwhelming amount of evidence now pointing to the failure of the traditional approach to medical education, the only surprise remains that the situation has persisted so long. The situation in secondary schools, in universities more generally, in some of the professions, and certainly in business and commerce, has developed to become much more effective educationally in the past half century, leaving medical education alone with its now discredited traditional approach.

Contemporary educational practice

Fortunately for medical education, contemporary medical education has risen to this challenge. The various chapters in this book testify to some exciting developments.

Chapter 1 outlines the basic principles on which the conference was founded. The intention of the organisers was to assemble invited experts in the fields of medicine and medical education to discuss the conference theme – learning in medicine. It would be inappropriate to lecture these people. Rather, they should be allowed, as far as possible, to decide the content of the conference for themselves. It should, within the bounds of possibility, be self directed. The organisers, for their part, would attempt to create a climate conducive to learning, and opportunities for people to interact. From then on, they would act as facilitators of the participants' learning.

Chapter 2 discusses lifelong self directed learning, which it suggests is crucial for medical people to develop the necessary "know how" for effective medical practice and for keeping up to date. A central attribute is the ability to reflect on one's practice and to learn through this. Lifelong self-directed learning can be accomplished in three ways: through the use of simulated patients, by peer and self review, and through the latest developments in medical informatics.

Chapter 3 takes some of these arguments further. Continuing medical education, that is the education of physicians that occurs after formal training, does not comprise distinct learning events but is a collective of many different elements. Central to this is the fact that physicians do indeed direct their own learning. Studies show that physicians adopting an innovation are influenced most by their colleagues and from their reading, and far less by attending conferences or through formalised CME programmes. The chapter discusses the linkage between life-long learning, continuing medical education, and the competence of physicians. The physicians' change study carried out in the United States of America suggests that forces for change help to clarify what should happen which directs the learning that is needed by exposing gaps in what the physician already knows, which in turn are filled through personal effort on the part of the physician.

Chapter 4 looks at how trainee doctors can acquire the skills they need to become self directed learners, and focuses on their relationship with their teachers. Medical learning occurs largely through in-service education. Meeting the needs of the health service necessarily has educational implications for the trainee doctor. Educational supervisors, normally the trainee's consultant or senior clinician, have the responsibility for establishing a supportive and constructive atmosphere within which learning can take place. Both teachers and learners bring their own agendas to any educational situation. Often there is a difference between what the learner wants to know and what the teacher sees the learner as needing to know. This distinction has to be resolved. Once learners have agreed on some learning objectives with their teachers they can then become self directed.

Chapter 5 describes how in Norway hospital consultants are being trained as educational counsellors, that is to provide professional development in their trainees by helping them integrate theoretical knowledge, practical experiences, and their personal values. It suggests that educational counsellors should encourage trainees to gain insight into, and an understanding of, the process of making decisions by making those problem solving processes explicit and by demonstrating what a professional might do and say. Central to this is the development by trainees of what is called a "practical theory" – that is to understand on what basis they carry out their professional practice. Consultants develop these counselling skills in workshops which themselves model the counselling process they are expected to adopt.

Chapter 6 discusses a model for change in a medical context – a check list rather than a recipe – which is based on doctors' accounts of change in which they have been involved. It is suggested that the bulk of the effort should be put into the preparatory stages, that is in establishing the need, ensuring one has sufficient power to act, designing the new scheme with consultation and publicity, and modifying it until it is the best that can be achieved within the constraints of time and effort available.

Chapter 7 describes how medical students can act as change agents in the development of their curricula since they are the people who most closely experience medical education and know about it from the inside. There are, of course, a number of problems in this suggestion. Medical students are short lived, and lack continuity. They are often not given inside information about the workings of the medical faculty or of the current curriculum, and frequently are not exposed to insights into education which these days even some of their teachers are receiving. Often, too, students are kept at arm's length by their teachers and frequently find themselves in an inferior position. Sometimes students are threatened by their teachers if they even attempt to question the status quo. Nevertheless students can make a useful contribution to educational change, and examples are given where this has occurred. Perhaps what is needed is a closer partnership between students and their teachers.

Chapter 8 discusses how information technology could have an impact on learning in general and medical knowledge transfer in particular. Many general practitioners are now using knowledge based systems, to transform how they work. These provide them with a very large (and potentially widely distributed) knowledge base which can support their decision making in consultations, and leave "an audit trail" for each consultation. One change is that this could make doctors' work more technical and less empathic, and medical education should be helping them develop their communication and decision making skills rather than asking them to acquire vast amounts of biomedical knowledge.

Chapter 9 reminds us that, in the face of exciting developments in information technology, reading and writing remain perhaps the most important learning tools in the study of medicine. Having said this, education has the potential for being utterly boring. The solution is to "let them see, feel, smell, hear, and taste" the subject, and in this way "to bring it alive". Education should be exciting, and fun, and should engage the learner's interest through questioning and controversy.

Chapter 11 describes the basis of the workshops which formed the bulk of the Oslo Conference, founded on the principles of self directed adult learning, where participants would interact with one another in small groups. It was recognised that there would be tensions between the two cultures represented at the conference. Medical people would require a clear agenda, while educationists would be happier with a more open one. These differences would need to be resolved. Participants would choose topics from a prearranged "menu" in the early stages of the conference, but later would determine their own topics and run their own workshops. Workshop leaders would act as facilitators; each workshop would have resource people to provide expertise and the workshop group would be the central learning vehicle. The fundamental aim was that individuals would gain their own personal insights, even if this took precedence over more concrete outcomes such as workshop reports.

From this brief review of the chapters in this book a number of principles emerge which underpin current developments in medical education. These are:

- The learner is the focus for current approaches to medical education.

- Learning itself is much more than merely acquiring information. It is qualitative not quantitative.
- The early stages of learning are crucially important. Learners need to establish for themselves, or agree with their teachers, some appropriate learning objectives.
- There is often a difference between what the learner wants to learn and what the teacher sees the learner as needing to learn. This must be resolved.
- Teachers need to develop skills for negotiating learning objectives.
- The climate in which education occurs is also important, and the teacher has a central role in this. The atmosphere created needs to be constructive and conducive to learning, and the learner's emotional state has a big influence on his or her motivation.
- Self-directed learning is predicated on the learner's ability to carry out self appraisal; to acknowledge his or her strengths and weaknesses, and through this to see the educational gaps.
- The teacher's role is to organise learning events and to facilitate learning, and not to act as the transmitter of information.
- These principles generalise across many fields. They can be seen in undergraduate and postgraduate medical education, in specialist training and in CME. They can even be applied to patient education.

Educational theories

What then has educational theory to say, and in what ways can this be of value to people working in medicine and medical education? For much of the first part of this century theories of learning were dominated by the work of two people – Pavlov in Russia, who described what he called classical conditioning, and Skinner, in North America, who described what he called operational learning. These two concepts have been applied in a number of human situations such as the prevention of enuresis in children, and programmed learning in education and training. Indeed, their work led to the development of an entire school of learning psychology called behaviourism. However, it was felt that just because animals and humans *could* learn this way, was it correct to say that they *did*? By the 1960s, a number of educational theorists were arguing against a behaviourist approach, and two broad themes emerged, both rooted in earlier work which had lain dormant for some forty or fifty years. The first takes a cognitive view of learning and the second sees it from a humanistic viewpoint.

1. Cognitive learning theory

Bartlett, in the 1930s, had been arguing that learning in general and memory in particular was a dynamic process (9). What we learnt, he suggested, was greatly influenced by how we learnt, which in turn was affected by what we already knew. When these ideas were taken up in the 1950s and 60s, learning became characterised as "information processing" (10). Incoming information is first received by the sensory organs, passed to a short term memory where it is processed, then stored in a long term memory. There is, however, a feedback mechanism: information already stored in long term memory has a central role in the processing that occurs in the short term memory.

The analogy often used is the way books are stored in a library (11). Newly acquired books are processed by the librarian using the classification and storage system currently being used. A library user wishing to retrieve a particular book, but knowing little about it, first goes to the appropriate index and thereby finds out where the book is located within the library. This is greatly helped by a cross referencing system. In human learning, we share new information in line with the already developed categories of our storage system, and effective retrieval occurs when we have "multiple roots of access" to the information which has already been stored.

Already, the information processing view of learning helps explain why parrot-fashion learning in undergraduate medical education is so grossly inefficient. Learning lists of facts is unlikely to process the information in terms of anything sensible, nor does it provide multiple roots of access to the stored information. As soon as you forget one item on the list, so you forget the remainder. Mnemonics are a good example. So long as you can remember the rhyme you can retrieve the important facts you have linked to it. Abstract information is arbitrarily attached to something which is memorable due to its vividness or nonsensical nature. Forget the rhyme and you can not retrieve the facts.

A further implication of the information processing theory of learning is that forgetting is not due to "fading" of the memory through some process of decay. Rather, forgetting is an "active" process, more likely to be due to not having known at the time the information was being stored the kinds of situations in which you were likely to need it in the future.

An important contribution to this information processing view of learning was made by Ausubel (12) who showed that learning was helped by the presence of what he called an "advanced organiser" which is some prior knowledge that helps us process the new inform-ation. Educationally this means we can help by ensuring that learners are "prepared" in some way.

In the 1970s, work in Gothenberg introduced the terms deep and surface processing to describe different levels of learning (13). Deep processing, it was suggested, refers to what happens when people attempt to understand the meaning of what they are learning, while surface processing occurs when people merely rote learn or memo-rise. These studies suggested that deep rather than surface processing led to educational success.

Studies in medical education confirm that students enter under-graduate courses with a deep processing orientation to their studying but, in traditional medical schools, quickly adopt a surface ap-proach, which is associated with poor academic performance (14). It has not, though, been shown that deep processing alone correlates with academic success. Rather, an elaborated approach, where stu-dents not only attempt to understand what they are learning but link together their knowledge into a kind of network, correlates with success (15). This kind of approach is more likely to be seen in prob-lem based medical schools, or in traditional medical schools where there are significant curricula features which encourage elaboration.

An extension of the information processing view of learning has been provided more recently by the work of Kolb (16), who speaks of learning occurring best through a cycle starting with actual experi-ence on which the learner reflects, derives some abstract principles from it, and applies those principles to new situations.

In a similar way, Schon argues that professional practice is based on unstated principles which involve the practitioner in a process he called "reflection in action" (17). Professionals he suggests in the course of their daily work hold a kind of dialogue with themselves in order to define the problems they face and begin to solve them, and carry out "on the spot experimentation" by subtly modifying their approach in ways that are untried and untested to meet the unique demands of each situation they have to deal with. He sug-gests, too, that professionals have the capacity to reflect on their practise, and to derive general principles that can guide their work, and in this way further elaborate their professional knowledge (18).

In much the same way, Polyani suggests that much professional knowledge is implicit and personal (19). Professionals may practice in similar ways yet their knowledge base can be quite different. Thus it would be quite wrong to assume that there is some core knowledge that underpins professional practice that can be transmitted through professional education. Rather, professionals must be allowed to create their own personal knowledge through the opportunities afforded by professional education.

From all of this it follows that professional learning is much more than merely being given information. It is concerned with the processing of information, and is highly dependent upon what we already know or have previously experienced. Knowledge getting is a process which is unique to each individual. Medical teachers can present the same information to a number of learners, yet each one will be processing it uniquely. Educators must recognise the difference between the information they think they have presented and the information that the learner has actually received and stored.

Effective information processing also depends on having some appropriate prior knowledge which needs to be broader and more inclusive than the specific information which has to be learnt. One implication is that the traditional "basic firsts" approach where theory is presented before practice is less efficient than when people first have some relevant practical experience, or are given some concrete example, which enables them to process effectively the abstract information, facts, and principles their teachers want them to learn.

Above all, effective learning is concerned with learners attempting to establish more and more complex networks of knowledge rather than storing information as discrete and separate entities. High quality learning, the basis for problem solving and professional thinking, results from "pulling things together", that is by constantly structuring and restructuring what we know into a more and more elaborated knowledge, which is the basis for problem solving and professional thinking.

2. Humanistic learning theory

A second thread of learning psychology has run through the twentieth century, and, like information processing, has its roots reaching back forty or fifty years. At this time, because of the introduction of automated work practices and repetitive business routines, occupational psychology, then known as industrial psychology, was beginning to become established. The idea of "time and motion" study was being developed (20). Employees were observed carrying out their everyday work in the workplace itself, and perhaps for the first time employment began to be seen from the point of view of the employee. Initially, these studies were carried out with the aim of improving worker efficiency. It soon became apparent, showever, that the analysis of job performance also helped employee training. Once skills had been observed and recorded, they could be broken down into their constituent parts, which could form the basis for training programmes.

From this it became clear that the working environment was an extremely important consideration. Employees subjected to excessive noise, heat, fumes, fatigue, etc., performed less well than those that were not, and improvements to the working environment led to improved efficiency.

In addition, a second major factor emerged, that of the morale of the workforce. It was discovered that the mere fact of altering the environmental conditions under which people worked led to increased efficiency. The conclusion was that the group being studied felt valued, and their self-esteem and motivation to work increased.

A third, and related, factor was also noted. Giving employees constructive feedback on their work increased their efficiency. Successful working practices that were praised led to enhanced performance. Poor working practices could be improved when they were critically appraised in a constructive manner that allowed employees to see the nature of their errors and how they could be rectified. Perhaps even more significantly, people improved their performance when they had the opportunity to observe the results of their own efforts and discover where they could make improvements. It was also found that trainees could quickly achieve higher levels of proficiency and more effective work practices when they were taught by people who themselves had been trained as trainers.

Although this "worker-centred" approach in an industrial setting directly connected work efficiencies with the employees' motivational state, it was not until the 1960s and 1970s that these concepts were applied to the world of education. The work of Rogers (21) was particularly significant here in developing the notion of learner-centred education. He argued that the learner should be the focus of education, and that the teacher's role was to provide support for learning to occur. For Rogers, learning was a "self actualising tendency". If learners were faced with the real problems of their existence learning would occur automatically because the learners would *want* to know how to solve the problems. The teacher's responsibility was to provide a supportive environment in which this could happen, that is, to facilitate learning.

Rogers' work closely followed on from the writings of Piaget (23) who showed that childrens' thinking passed through a series of developmental stages, leading in the teenage years to a shift from concrete to abstract thought. Perry (24), working with college students, demonstrated that development did not stop there. He suggested that young adults continued with their intellectual development. He suggested that students begin by seeing knowledge as being either right or wrong, and pass to a position when they see that truth is dependent upon the context in which the knowledge is located. Ultimately, they commit themselves to a particular view of knowledge that both fits their own thinking and helps determine it. The teacher's role, according to Perry, is to help students pass through this developmental period, and in particular to help them see the relativistic nature of knowledge. However, Perry acknowledges that this transition is sometimes difficult and even painful for students, and that teachers need considerable patience in helping students grapple with their uncertainties.

The role of the individual learner was further developed by Knowles (22) in relation to adult learners. He introduced the term "self directed learning" where learners are encouraged to set their own learning objectives and, together with others, seek their own solutions to their problems.

In many ways, all of this work signalled a political shift of emphasis in education. The teacher was no longer dominant, learning became more important than teaching, and the learner's state of mind more significant than the teacher's.

This shift emphasised the relationship between our intellectual and emotional states of mind. Maslow (25), for example, had suggested that we have a "hierarchy of needs". We must address our physiological needs first. Once these are met we must satisfy our social needs. Only then can we address our intellectual needs. For Maslow, education should be concerned not just with *what* we are teaching, but *why* we are teaching it. Schools, he said, "should be helping the children to look within themselves, and from this self knowledge derive a set of values".

Brown (26), too, emphasises these links in what he terms confluent education. He says, "it should be apparent that there is no learning without some sort of feeling, and there are no feelings without the mind being somehow involved".

At about the same time, considerable interest developed into the ways in which learners could work together as a group, with or without a teacher being present, and techniques of small group learning began to be developed (27), promoting cooperative and collaborative learning activities rather than the competitive and coercive ones seen more commonly in traditional approaches to education.

A synthesis

We have seen, then, how two strands of educational enquiry have developed over the earlier parts of this century. The first sees learning as the processing of information; the second looks at the learner's context referring both to what is going on inside the learners and the environment surrounds them. What these two threads clearly show is that education has two facets. First, education should be concerned with ensuring that someone is *able* to work well, and second, that that person *wants* to work well. One is concerned with competence. It is about making sure that the person *can* do the job. The other, which is equally important, concerns the person's motivational state, the desire to do the job to the best of his or her ability. When we consider that education is concerned (in part) with "preparing" people, we need to recognise that we are using the term "prepared" in both these senses simultaneously. Put another way, as educators we should ask: Are people as a result of our education prepared to do the job in the sense of being competent to do it to the best of their ability, and are they willing to do it to the best of their ability?

A theory of medical education

Perhaps the failure of medical education in the past to provide optimal conditions for learning to take place has been because there has been no appropriate theory of medical education. Now would seem to be an entirely appropriate opportunity to develop such a theory.

Drawing on the theoretical and practical descriptions presented in this book, the following theory of medical education is proposed:

In medical education, people will learn best when they are helped to reflect on practice, to identify the strengths and weaknesses within it, to identify educational objectives for themselves as a result, to deal with these objectives satisfactorily, from a cognitive as well as an emotional perspective, to evaluate their progress in meeting them, and as a result to apply what they have learnt in their own practice. The teacher's role is to provide an environment in which this can occur, to monitor the learner's progress, to provide constructive feedback as appropriate, and to intervene appropriately as necessary in order to facilitate the learning that is occurring.

In practical terms, two factors need to be clarified in order to operationalise this theory. These are 1) the educational setting, and 2) the roles of the various people involved.

1. The educational setting

For appropriate learning to occur, the educational setting requires three features as shown in Figure 1. These comprise: (i) establishing an appropriate context for learning, (ii) making available the necessary information, and (iii) providing opportunities for effective learning to take place.

(i) The context for learning
Learning takes place in a context. The task for the educator is to ensure that that context is an appropriate one. The learning context can be considered from two points of view: *the context within the learner*, and *the context outside the learner.*

Internal learning context
The internal context of the learner comprises not just his or her cognitive state but also the physiological emotional state.

To pay attention to the internal cognitive state means, as Ausubel puts it, finding out what the learner already knows, and proceeding from there (12). This includes assessing the learner's knowledge, the experiences the learner has had, and the analytical frameworks for understanding that the learner has already developed. Often, though, learners do not know what they already know, and may need to be helped to recognise their own starting point for learning. This is where the concept of reflection is so important.

Within the learner, the physiological and emotional context should be a satisfactory one. The task of clarifying it, however, is not always easy. Although most learners are aware of hunger, tiredness, discomfort, etc., often they have not learnt to express their feelings. Emotions can facilitate or inhibit learning; therefore, it is essential

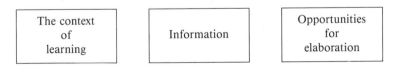

Figure 1. The contextual learning model (8)

that the teacher assists the learner in reaching a high degree of self awareness about his or her internal context. This is especially important in clinical teaching as the students or doctors are often faced with situations that provoke emotional responses. If the learning climate does not provide ample opportunity for students deliberately to face and integrate their cognitive and emotional states, inappropriate cognitive and emotional coping strategies may ensue. These will not only affect the students' or doctors' ability to learn, but may also represent a threat to the health. It is therefore essential that expression of feelings are valued and that they are met in a non-judgemental way. Clinical practice implies living with uncertainties. The medical student and doctor must learn to live with them, and to feel comfortable doing so.

External learning context
The external learning context concerns the things going on around the learner that ensure effective learning will take place. This includes environmental factors regarding the location, for instance, the degree of comfort or distraction. The external context can, of course, be deliberately manipulated by the teacher. For example, learning can be enhanced when learners are presented with some relevant concrete experience very early on in any learning sequence. This could involve the learner's participation in an activity specially devised for the occasion, or some involvement in routine practices. It might also involve providing the learner with some appropriate example or illustration to form a basis of the subsequent learning. This can be seen in *problem-based learning*, where the problem, even if a "paper case", provides a concrete beginning for the learning process. In on-the-job learning, the context comprises what the learner is actually doing or has just completed.

(ii) Information
The second feature of the educational setting as shown in Figure 1 is the availability of appropriate information. By definition, this information will be more abstract than the concrete context already established. On its own, that is in the absence of an appropriate learning context, this information is likely to carry very little meaning for the learner. It will be novel. Care needs to be taken to ensure that the information made available or presented to the learner at this point has a clear relationship to the learning context already established. For example, in problem based learning, the nature of the problem that forms the context for learning and the information

made available subsequently has to be a matter of careful consideration on the part of the teacher and curriculum planners. Similarly, too, in experiential learning, care must be taken that the generalisations that the learner makes concerning the experience being reflected upon have a clear relationship with that experience. Put another way, there is an issue here concerning relevance. The information derived by, made available for, or presented to the learner must be relevant to the learner's context.

In practice, curriculum planners will simultaneously consider the learning context and the information being made available. Clearly, though, there are dangers that the context and the information may not match, or, perhaps more worrying, that the learner does not recognise the mismatch and wrongly connects theory and practice.

Paradoxically, the presentation of information *after* the establishment of the learning context is the complete opposite of how most medical education is structured. Traditionally, facts are presented before their application. Theory comes before practice. The preclinical course precedes the clinical course. All the examples of good practice presented in this book, and all the theories of education presented earlier in this chapter, suggest that the traditional approach, while rational at one level, is educationally inappropriate. Practice should precede, or be closely interrelated with, theory. We learn theory best through its practical application.

(iii) Opportunities for elaboration
The third element of the educational setting shown in Figure 1 concerns opportunities for elaborating (15). Even if an appropriate context for learning has been established, and appropriate information has been made available, there remains the need for the learner to make the link between the information and the context, that is between theory and practice. This is a task which only the learner can perform. The teacher cannot do it for the learner. Learning is a journey of discovery, and a very personal one. However, the learner may not make the connections automatically or accurately. The teacher, while being unable to learn *for* the student, can, and often must, arrange the educational setting so that the learner has the opportunity to learn in this way.

Opportunities for elaboration could occur in discussion between the teacher and the learner, provided the teacher adopts a role that encourages exploration by the learner. Alternatively, appropriate opportunities can occur in group discussion, private study, through computer-assisted learning, and even while revising for examinations.

The kind of learning that the learner engages in is also very important. Gaining knowledge is much more than merely acquiring information. It is an active process on the part of the learner that takes information from the outside and makes it personal to the learner. Knowledge is not the quantitative accumulation of facts but the qualitative transformation of information into an elaborate structured entity. Knowledge is greater than the sum of its parts.

Again, the good teacher encourages the learner to do this. Some learners may do it quite naturally. Others may have to learn how to elaborate their knowledge. In the case of experiential learning, elaboration occurs when learners generalise from the specific instance on which they are reflecting to new situations they want to try out. In problem-based learning, it can happen when learners engage in the act of problem solving by utilizing the knowledge they have gained in the light of one problem and applying it in the solution of new ones. Evaluation is also evident when learners make intuitive leaps in their understanding. That is when they gain sudden insights, and when "things fit together". Frequently these experiences are highly motivating for learners, and they provide the all important intrinsic rewards associated with "learning for its own sake".

2. The roles of the people involved in education

Curriculum planners, teachers, and even learners themselves could learn effectively by ensuring that the three features of the model presented above are in place, for everyone involved: learners, teachers, and people responsible for the institution itself.

(i) Learners

It is clear that the learner must be an active participant in the learning process. He or she must learn how to reflect on experience, and how to observe actual situations so as to provide a necessary "advance organiser" for learning to take place. Learners, too, may need to learn how to link theory and practice, and how to apply their knowledge "beyond the information given". Moreover, learners may need to learn how to seek help from their colleagues and from their teachers.

Not all learners though are effective learners, and some will need help. The approaches described in Chapters 4 and 5 indicate ways in which this can happen, and other possibilities could be explored.

(ii) Teachers

Teachers, of course have a number of responsibilities for ensuring education is as effective as possible. They need to establish the educational setting shown in Figure 1. The context for learning may well need to be created specifically, appropriate information or resource material may need to be made available, and teachers must ensure that opportunities occur for handling the information appropriately.

In addition, the teacher should monitor the learner's progress and intervene to facilitate effective learning. This is likely to involve the teacher in a number of activities not commonly found in traditional teaching. As seen in Chapter 4, teachers should allow learners to agree with them on their learning objectives. Teachers must recognize and resolve the distinction between what the learner wants to know and what the teacher believes the learner needs to know.

Intervention of this kind means teachers employ certain skills such as active listening. Here the learner has the opportunity to say what is in his or her mind. Teachers hold back from saying what they believe they have to say. As well active listening involves showing an interest in what the other person is saying, utilising non-verbal signals such as eye contact, nodding, looking engaged in the conversation, and using open rather than closed questions, for example, "What did you do in that situation?" rather than "Did you do such and such?".

Very importantly, learning is facilitated when the teacher gives the learner constructive feedback. This means praising the learner's successes, and pointing out the errors, particularly by saying why something was inappropriate and what might have been better. Even more important, the teacher should encourage the learner to self appraise his or her own performance.

Teachers have a natural urge to tell learners what they know and show them what they can do. This has to be suppressed as much as possible for the teacher to facilitate learning. Related to this is the difficulty some teachers have when a learner appears slow at grasping what seems very clear to them. Rogers emphasises the importance of what he calls "unconditional positive regard" for the learner, including trying to understand what difficulties there are in the subject from the learner's point of view. One of the most difficult aspects of being a teacher is not to know something, yet this is precisely what a teacher must try to do.

(iii) Institutions

The people in charge of educational institutions also have a responsibility. Education can be valued in some very practical ways, for example by providing the necessary resources, such as allocating specific time for educational planning and preparation, by providing time for interactions between teachers and learners, and by allowing time in which learning can take place over and above the learner's other commitments such as attending formal teaching sessions, or carrying out routine clinical work. There is a need to protect time for education, which may mean covering work that would have been carried out by the people who are engaging in education. In particular, they should value education in its own right. Generally in medical education this does not happen. Often, research comes higher than education in people's estimation, particularly regarding funding and staff promotion.

The importance of teaching as a skilled activity also needs to be recognised. Medical teachers are rarely trained to teach. It is crucial that they receive adequate and appropriate training. Teachers are often senior members of a profession, and teacher training should be seen as part of their continuing education. Closely linked with teacher training should be the regular appraisal of teaching. As part of this, teachers should be encouraged to develop teaching portfolios to demonstrate the quality of their teaching in much the same way that lists of publications indicate a researcher's output.

Teacher appraisal should have at least four functions. It should provide an opportunity for teachers to gain insight into their own teaching abilities; it should motivate teachers to want to teach as well as possible; it should provide opportunities for teachers to identify their weaknesses and to clarify their continuing needs for teacher training; and it should act as a regulatory mechanism. Not everybody can be expected to teach well. Inevitably, some people will teach badly, despite teacher training, and they should be encouraged to work in areas other than in teaching.

Closely linked with the appraisal of teachers should be a reward system which gives value to teaching. Appointments, confirmation of posts, and promotions for anyone working in medical education should all involve a recognition of the teaching carried out by the individual. In future, it is not at all unlikely that performance related pay will become more common. Good teachers should be rewarded for their efforts.

Finally, the institution should ensure that education is satisfactorily audited. In the past, education has been haphazard and unregulated. It has merely "happened". There has been little attempt to record the education that is taking place, let alone evaluate its effectiveness. This situation is unlikely to be allowed to continue much longer. One problem is that education is an extremely "soft" endeavour. Apart from formal teaching, it is difficult to identify when and where it is actually occurring, or to "measure" in some objective way its attributes. Nevertheless, attempts have been made to audit education, and considerably more effort now needs to be put into this.

Conclusion

In this chapter an attempt has been made to pull together a number of threads running through this book. It began with a review of traditional medical education and some of the problems created by it. Alternative educational approaches, as described within this book, were then summarised. Following this, educational theories were reviewed, and two threads emerged: a cognitive view of learning concerning the way in which humans process information, and a humanistic view of learning which emphasises the learners' external and internal environment.

This led to the proposal of a theory for medical education which emphasizes the importance of learners agreeing with their teachers their educational objectives, and being helped by teachers to achieve them themselves. It was suggested this is possible if the educational setting comprises three elements: the context; the information; and the opportunities for handling that information. This has implications for learners, teachers, and institutions.

The theory proposed here explains the weaknesses in the traditional educational system, as well as accounts for the apparent successes of the alternative approaches described throughout this book. But any competent theory needs to be predictive. Can it be said that education based on this theory leads to better educational outcomes?

One educational innovation which has had a significant impact on medical education in the past twenty years or so, problem-based learning, appears to meet the conditions of the proposed theory. So too does the educational approach described in chapter 4 for training medical teachers. More objective evidence is required though before it can be said that the theory has created a better educational outcome, and further results are awaited before it can be said that this theory has strong predictive power.

This contextual learning theory of medical education is, therefore, proposed as a basis for development in both undergraduate and postgraduate medicine. People establishing educational programmes could take it as the basis for evaluating existing programmes and for planning new ones. Their experience in doing so should be shared as widely as possible if a coherent and competent theory is to be established.

References

1. Coles CR. Diabetes education: theories of practice. Practical Diabetes 1989; 6: 199-202.
2. Berne E. Games people play. Harmondsworth: Penguin Books, 1964.
3. Becker HS, Geer B, Hughes, EC, Strauss A. Boys in white. Chicago: University of Chicago Press, 1961.
4. Simpson MA. Medical Education: A critical approach. London: Butterworth, 1972.
5. Maddison DC. What's wrong with medical education, Med Educ 1978; 12: 97-106.
6. Holm U. Empati i läkar-pasientrelationen. Acta Univ Ups. Upps Stud Educ 24. Stockholm: Almquist & Wiksell, 1985.
7. Coles, CR. Differences between conventional and problem-based curricula in their students' approaches to studying. Med Educ 1985; 19:
8. Coles, CR. A study of the relationships between curriculum and learning in undergraduate medical education. PhD thesis. Southampton: University of Southampton, 1985.
9. Bartlett RC. Remembering. Cambridge: Cambridge University Press, 1932.
10. Klatsky R. Human Memory: Structures and Processes, 2nd Edition. San Francisco: W H Freeman & Co, 1980.
11. Broadbent DE. Cognitive psychology and education. Brit J Ed Psych 1975; 45: 162-76.
12. Ausubel DP, Novak JS, Hanesian H. Educational Psychology: A Cognitive View, 2nd Edition. New York: Holt, Rinehart and Winston, 1978.
13. Marton F, Saljo R. On qualitative differences in learning II – outcome as a function of the learner's conception of the task. Brit J Ed Psych 1976; 46: 115-27.
14. Newble D, Entwistle N J, Hejka E J, Jolley B, Whelan G. Towards the identification of student learning problems: the development of a diagnostic inventory. Med Educ 1988; 22: 518-26.
15. Coles CR. Elaborated learning in undergraduate medical education. Med Educ 1990; 24: 14-22.
16. Kolb DA. Experiential learning: experience as a source of learning and development. Engelwood Cliffs: Prentice Hall 1984.
17. Schön DA . The reflective practitioner: how practitioners think in action. San Francisco: Jossey-Bass, 1983.
18. Schön DA. Educating the reflective practitioner: towards a new design for teaching and learning in the professions. San Francisco: Jossey Bass, 1987.
19. Polyani M. Personal Knowledge. London: Routledge & Kegan, 1958.
20. Munn NL. Psychology: The fundamental of human adjustment. London: Harrap, 1956.
21. Rogers CR. Freedom to learn. Colombus: Merril, 1969.

22. Knowles MS. The Modern Practice of Adult Education. Androgogy vs Pedagogy. New York: Association Press, 1970.
23. Piaget J. Intellectual development from adolescence. Human Development 1972;15: 1-12.
24. Perry WG. Forms of intellectual and ethical development in the college years: a scheme. New York: Holt Rinehart & Winston, 1970.
25. Maslow A. The farther reaches of human nature. Harmondsworth: Penguin Books, 1973.
26. Brown GI. Human teaching for human learning. New York: Gestalt Journal Press, 1990.
27. Walton HJ. Small group methods in medical teaching. Medical Education Booklet 1. Dundee: Association for the Study of Medical Education, 1973.

Contributors

Philip Bashook
American Board of Medical Specialties
Chicago, Illinois, USA

Guttorm Brattebø
Hammerfest Hospital
Hammerfest, Norway

Colin Coles
University of Southampton, Faculty of Medicine
Southampton, UK

Janet Grant
Joint Centre for Educational Research and
Development in Medicine
London, UK

Hans Asbjørn Holm
The Norwegian Medical Association
Lysaker, Norway

Penny Jennett
University of Calgary, Medical Faculty
Calgary, Canada

Kirsten Lycke
The Norwegian Medical Association
Lysaker, Norway

Peter Prichard
UK-Nordic Medical Education Trust
Oxfordshire, UK

Richard Smith
British Medical Journal
London, UK